Lecture Notes

Dermat

Robin Graham-Brown

BSc, MB BS (Lond), FRCP, FRCPCH
Consultant Dermatologist
University Hospitals of Leicester
Honorary Senior Lecturer in Dermatology
University of Leicester

Tony Burns

MB BS (Lond), FRCP
Emeritus Consultant Dermatologist
The Leicester Royal Infirmary, Leicester

Ninth Edition

2013 → Plymouth

First published 1965
Second edition 1969
Third edition 1973
Fourth edition 1977
Fifth edition 1983
Sixth edition 1990
Seventh edition 1996
Eighth edition 2002
Ninth edition 2007

2 2007

Library of Congress Cataloging-in-Publication Data
Graham-Brown, R. A. C. (Robin A. C.)
    Lecture notes. Dermatology / Robin Graham-Brown, Tony Burns. – 9th ed.
        p. ; cm.
    Rev. ed. of: Lectures notes on dermatology. 8th ed. 2002.
    Includes bibliographical references and index.
    ISBN 978-1-4051-3977-9 (alk. paper)
        1. Dermatology–Outlines, syllabi, etc.   2. Skin–Diseases–Outlines, syllabi, etc.   I. Burns,
Tony, FRCP. II. Graham-Brown, R. A. C. (Robin A. C.). Lectures notes on dermatology. III. Title.
IV. Title: Dermatology.
    [DNLM: 1. Skin Diseases.   WR 140 G742L 2007]
    RL74.3.G73 2007
    616.5–dc22

2006020169

A catalogue record for this title is available from the British Library

Set in 8/12 Stone Serif by SNP Best-set Typesetter Ltd., Hong Kong
Printed and bound in Singapore by Fabulous Printers Pte Ltd

Commissioning Editor: Martin Sugden
Editorial Assistant: Eleanor Bonnet
Development Editor: Hayley Salter
Production Controller: Debbie Wyer

For further information on Blackwell Publishing, visit our website:
http://www.blackwellpublishing.com

Dewey no.	Subject headings
616.5	dermatology
Location	Abstract
CHSW	March 2008
3 Week	Order details
1 Week	
LUO	P0080779/Q LC £19-05
Reference	

Contents

Preface

In this, the ninth edition of *Lecture Notes: Dermatology*, we have updated the text with particular regard to recent advances in the knowledge of skin diseases and developments in therapy. Numerous tables of salient points provide ready reference but, as in previous editions, we have attempted to create a 'user-friendly' readability.

We hope that the book will be of value not only to medical students, but also to general practitioners, and nurses involved in the care of dermatology patients. We also hope that exposure to *Lecture Notes: Dermatology* will stimulate a deeper interest in this important medical specialty.

Robin Graham-Brown
Tony Burns

Acknowledgements

We are indebted to the late Dr Imrich Sarkany, and to Charles Calnan, under whose guidance we both learned dermatology. We are also grateful to all the medical students who, over many years, have reminded us of the importance of clarity in communication, and that teaching should be a stimulating and enjoyable experience for everyone concerned. Finally, we thank the staff at Blackwell Publishing who have helped us through the editing and production stages.

Chapter 1

Structure and function of the skin, hair and nails

Skin, skin is a wonderful thing,
Keeps the outside out and the inside in.

It is essential to have some background knowledge of the normal structure and function of any organ before you can hope to understand the abnormal. Skin is the icing on the anatomical cake, it is the decorative wrapping paper, and without it not only would we all look rather unappealing, but a variety of unpleasant physiological phenomena would bring about our demise. You have probably never contemplated your skin a great deal, except in the throes of narcissistic admiration, or when it has been blemished by some disorder, but hopefully by the end of this first chapter you will have been persuaded that it is quite a remarkable organ, and that you are lucky to be on such intimate terms with it.

Skin structure

The skin is composed of two layers, the epidermis and the dermis (Fig. 1.1). The epidermis, which is the outer layer, and its appendages (hair, nails, sebaceous glands and sweat glands) are derived from the embryonic ectoderm. The dermis is of mesodermal origin.

The epidermis

The epidermis is a stratified squamous epithelium, with several well-defined layers. The principal cell type is known as a *keratinocyte*. Keratinocytes, pro-duced by cell division in the deepest layer of the epidermis (basal layer), are carried towards the skin surface where they are shed. In health, the rate of production of cells matches the rate of loss, so that epidermal thickness is constant. Epidermal kinetics are controlled by a number of growth stimulators and inhibitors. The time taken for a cell to pass from the basal layer to the surface in normal skin (epidermal turnover time or transit time) is around 50 days, but this is much shorter in psoriasis.

As keratinocytes pass towards the skin surface, they undergo a complex series of morphological and biochemical changes known as *terminal differentiation* (keratinization) to produce the surface layer of tightly packed dead cells (stratum corneum or horny layer). So-called *intermediate filaments*, present in the cytoplasm of epithelial cells, are a major component of the cytoskeleton. They contain a group of fibrous proteins known as keratins, each of which is the product of a separate gene. Mutations in these genes are responsible for certain diseases. Pairs of keratins are characteristic of certain cell types and tissues, and K5/K14 are characteristic of stratified squamous epithelia. Epidermal basal cells express K5 and K14, but K1 and K10 are also expressed during differentiation in the suprabasal layers.

As cells reach the higher layers of the epidermis, filaments aggregate under the influence of a protein known as *filaggrin*, derived from its precursor

1

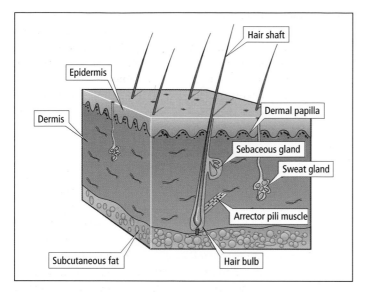

Figure 1.1 The structure of the skin.

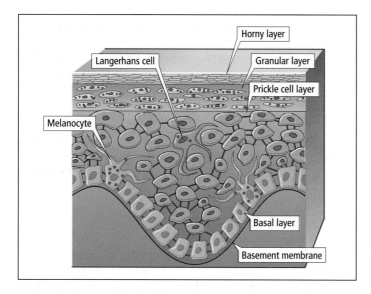

Figure 1.2 The epidermis.

profilaggrin, present in *keratohyalin granules* that constitute the granules in the granular layer.

Other components of the differentiation process include production of a *cornified cell envelope* (that has important mechanical and barrier functions) around cells in the stratum corneum, and the production of lipids.

Look at the layers more closely (Fig. 1.2). The basal layer, which is 1–3 cells thick, is anchored to a basement membrane (see below) that lies be-tween the epidermis and dermis. Interspersed among the basal cells are melanocytes—large dendritic cells derived from the neural crest—which are responsible for melanin pigment production. Melanocytes contain cytoplasmic organelles called melanosomes, in which melanin is synthesized from tyrosine. The melanosomes migrate along the dendrites of the melanocytes, and are transferred to the keratinocytes in the prickle cell layer. In white people, the melanosomes are grouped together in membrane-bound *melanosome complexes*, and they gradually degenerate as the keratinocytes move towards the surface of the skin. The skin of black people contains the same number of melanocytes as that of white people, but the melanosomes are larger, remain separate and persist through the full thickness of the epidermis. The main stimulus to melanin production is ultraviolet (UV) radiation. Melanin protects the cell nuclei in the epidermis from the harmful effects of UV radiation. A sun tan is a natural protective mechanism, not some God-given cosmetic boon created so that you can impress the neighbours on your return from an exotic foreign trip! Unfortunately, this does not appear to be appreciated by the pale, pimply lager-swilling advert for British manhood who dashes onto the beach in Ibiza and flash-fries himself to lobster thermidor on day one of his annual holiday.

Skin neoplasia is extremely uncommon in dark-skinned races because their skin is protected from UV damage by the large amounts of melanin it contains. However, individuals with albinism are predisposed to skin cancer because their production of melanin is impaired and they are therefore without its protective influence.

Above the basal layer is the prickle cell/spinous layer. This acquires its name from the spiky appearance produced by intercellular bridges (desmosomes) that connect adjacent cells. Important in cell–cell adhesion are several protein components of desmosomes, including cadherins (desmogleins and desmocollins) and plakins. Production of these is genetically controlled, and abnormalities have been detected in some human diseases.

Scattered throughout the prickle cell layer are Langerhans cells. These dendritic cells contain characteristic racquet-shaped 'Birbeck' granules. Langerhans cells are probably modified macrophages, which originate in the bone marrow and migrate to the epidermis. They are the first line of immunological defence against environmental antigens (see below).

Above the prickle cell layer is the granular layer, which is composed of flattened cells containing the darkly staining keratohyalin granules. Also present in the cytoplasm of cells in the granular layer are organelles known as lamellar granules (Odland bodies). These contain lipids and enzymes, and they discharge their contents into the intercellular spaces between the cells of the granular layer and stratum corneum—providing the equivalent of 'mortar' between the cellular 'bricks', and contributing to the barrier function of the epidermis.

The cells of the stratum corneum are flattened, keratinized cells that are devoid of nuclei and cytoplasmic organelles. Adjacent cells overlap at their margins, and this locking together of cells, together with intercellular lipid, forms a very effective barrier. The stratum corneum varies in thickness according to the region of the body. It is thickest on the palms of the hands and soles of the feet. The stratum corneum cells are gradually abraded by daily wear and tear. If you bathe after a period of several days' avoidance of water (a house without central heating, in mid-winter, somewhere in the high latitudes, is ideal for this experiment), you will note that as you towel yourself you are rubbing off small balls of keratin – which has built up because of your insanitary habits. When a plaster cast is removed from a fractured limb after several weeks *in situ*, there is usually a thick layer of surface keratin, the removal of which provides hours of absorbing occupational therapy.

Figure 1.3 shows the histological appearance of normal epidermis.

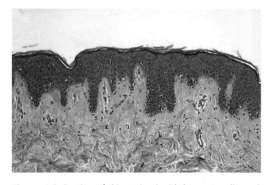

Figure 1.3 Section of skin stained with haematoxylin and eosin, showing the appearance of a normal epidermis. 'Rete ridges' (downward projections of the epidermis) interdigitate with 'dermal papillae' (upward projections of the dermis).

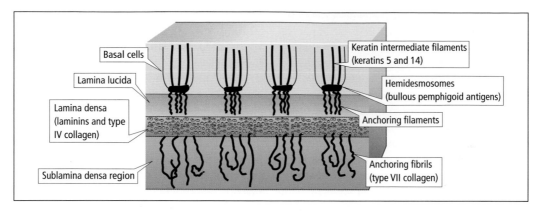

Figure 1.4 Structure of the basement membrane zone.

The basement membrane zone

This is composed of a number of layers, and it is important to have some knowledge of these as certain diseases are related to abnormalities in the layers. The basic structure is shown in Figure 1.4. Basal keratinocytes are attached by *hemidesmosomes* to the epidermal side of the membrane, and these have an important role in maintaining adhesion between the epidermis and dermis. The basement membrane is composed of three layers: lamina lucida (uppermost), lamina densa and sublamina densa region. A system of *anchoring filaments* connects hemidesmosomes to the lamina densa, and *anchoring fibrils*, which are closely associated with collagen in the upper dermis, connect the lamina densa to the dermis beneath.

The hemidesmosome/anchoring filament region contains autoantigens targeted by autoantibodies in immunobullous disorders (including bullous pemphigoid, pemphigoid gestationis, cicatricial pemphigoid and linear IgA bullous dermatosis; see Chapter 14)—hence the subepidermal location of blistering in these disorders.

The inherited blistering diseases (Chapter 14) occur as a consequence of mutations in genes responsible for components of the basement membrane zone. For example, epidermolysis bullosa simplex, in which splits occur in the basal keratinocytes, is related to mutations in genes coding for keratins 5 and 14, and dystrophic epidermolysis bullosa, in which blistering occurs immediately below the lamina densa, is related to mutations in a gene coding for type VII collagen, the major component of anchoring fibrils.

Epidermal appendages

The eccrine and apocrine sweat glands, the hair and sebaceous glands, and the nails constitute the epidermal appendages.

Eccrine sweat glands

Eccrine sweat glands are important in body temperature regulation. A human has between two and three million eccrine sweat glands covering almost all the body surface. They are particularly numerous on the palms of the hands and soles of the feet. Each consists of a secretory coil deep in the dermis, and a duct that conveys the sweat to the surface. Eccrine glands secrete water, electrolytes, lactate, urea and ammonia. The secretory coil produces isotonic sweat, but sodium chloride is reabsorbed in the duct so that sweat reaching the surface is hypotonic. Patients suffering from cystic fibrosis have defective resorption of sodium chloride, and rapidly become salt depleted in a hot environment. Eccrine sweat glands are innervated by the sympathetic nervous system, but the neurotransmitter is acetylcholine.

Apocrine sweat glands

Apocrine sweat glands are found principally in the axillae and anogenital region. Specialized apocrine glands include the wax glands of the ear and the milk glands of the breast. Apocrine glands are also composed of a secretory coil and a duct, but the duct opens into a hair follicle, not directly onto the surface of the skin. Apocrine glands produce an oily secretion containing protein, carbohydrate, ammonia and lipid. These glands become active at puberty, and secretion is controlled by adrenergic nerve fibres. Pungent axillary body odour (axillary bromhidrosis) is the result of the action of bacteria on apocrine secretions. In some animals, apocrine secretions are important sexual attractants, but the average human armpit provides a different type of overwhelming olfactory experience.

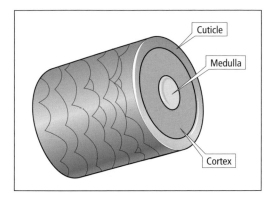

Figure 1.5 The structure of hair.

Hair

Hairs grow out of tubular invaginations of the epidermis known as follicles, and a hair follicle and its associated sebaceous glands are referred to as a 'pilosebaceous unit'. There are three types of hair: fine, soft *lanugo* hair is present *in utero* and is shed by the eighth month of fetal life; *vellus* hair is the fine downy hair which covers most of the body except those areas occupied by terminal hair; thick and pigmented *terminal* hair occurs on the scalp, eyebrows and eyelashes before puberty—after puberty, under the influence of androgens, secondary sexual terminal hair develops from vellus hair in the axillae and pubic region, and on the trunk and limbs in men. On the scalp, the reverse occurs in male-pattern balding—terminal hair becomes vellus hair under the influence of androgens. In men, terminal hair on the body usually increases in amount as middle age arrives, and hairy ears and nostrils, and bushy eyebrows are puzzling accompaniments of advancing years. One struggles to think of any biological advantage conferred by exuberant growth of hair in these sites.

Hair follicles extend into the dermis at an angle (Fig. 1.1). A small bundle of smooth muscle fibres, the arrector pili muscle, is attached to the side of the follicle. Arrector pili muscles are supplied by adrenergic nerves, and are responsible for the erection of hairs in the cold or during emotional stress ('goose flesh', 'goose pimples', horripilation). The duct of the sebaceous gland enters the follicle just above the point of attachment of the arrector pili

muscle. At the lower end of the follicle is the hair bulb, part of which, the hair matrix, is a zone of rapidly dividing cells that is responsible for the formation of the hair shaft. Hair pigment is produced by melanocytes in the hair bulb. Cells produced in the hair bulb become densely packed, elongated and arranged parallel to the long axis of the hair shaft. They gradually become keratinized as they ascend in the hair follicle.

The main part of each hair fibre is the cortex, which is composed of keratinized spindle-shaped cells (Fig. 1.5). Terminal hairs have a central core known as the medulla, consisting of specialized cells that contain air spaces. Covering the cortex is the cuticle, a thin layer of cells that overlap like the tiles on a roof, with the free margins of the cells pointing towards the tip of the hair. The cross-sectional shape of hair varies with body site and race. Negroid hair is distinctly oval in cross-section, and pubic, beard and eyelash hairs have an oval cross-section in all racial types. Caucasoid hair is moderately elliptical in cross-section and Mongoloid hair is circular.

The growth of each hair is cyclical—periods of active growth alternate with resting phases. After each period of active growth (anagen) there is a short transitional phase (catagen), followed by a resting phase (telogen), after which the follicle reactivates, a new hair is produced, and the old hair is shed. The duration of these cyclical phases depends on the age of the individual and the location of the follicle on the body. The duration of anagen in a scalp follicle is genetically determined, and ranges from 2 to more than 5 years. This is why some women can grow hair down to their ankles, whereas most have a much shorter maximum length. Scalp hair catagen lasts about 2 weeks and telogen from 3 to 4 months. The daily growth rate of scalp hair is approximately 0.45 mm. The activity of each follicle is independent of that of its neighbours, which is fortunate, because if follicular activity was synchronized, as it is in some animals, we would be subject to periodic moults, thus adding another dimension to life's rich tapestry. At any one time, approximately 85% of scalp hairs are in anagen, 1% in catagen and 14% in telogen. The average number of hairs shed daily is 100. In areas other than the scalp anagen is relatively short—this is also fortunate, because if it was not so, we would all be kept busy clipping eyebrows, eyelashes and nether regions.

It is a myth that shaving increases the rate of growth of hair and that it encourages the development of 'thicker' hair; nor does hair continue growing after death—shrinkage of soft tissues around the hair produces this illusion.

Human hair colour is principally dependent on two types of melanin: eumelanins in black and brown hair, and phaeomelanins in red, auburn and blond hair.

Greying of hair (canities) is the result of a decrease in tyrosinase activity in the melanocytes of the hair bulb. The age of onset of greying is genetically determined, but other factors may be involved such as autoimmunity—premature greying of the hair is a recognized association of pernicious anaemia. The phenomenon of 'going white overnight', usually attributed to a severe fright, is physically impossible. It is, however, possible to 'go white' over a period of a few days as a result of selective loss of remaining pigmented hairs in someone who has extensive grey hair—this occurs in one type of alopecia areata.

Sebaceous glands

Sebaceous glands are found everywhere on the skin apart from the hands and feet. They are particularly numerous and prominent on the head and neck, the chest and the back. Sebaceous glands are part of the pilosebaceous unit, and their lipid-rich product (sebum) flows through a duct into the hair follicle. They are holocrine glands—sebum is produced by disintegration of glandular cells rather than an active secretory process. Modified sebaceous glands that open directly on the surface are found on the eyelids, lips, nipples, glans penis and prepuce, and the buccal mucosa (Fordyce spots).

Sebaceous glands are prominent at birth, under the influence of maternal hormones, but atrophy soon after, and do not enlarge again until puberty. Enlargement of the glands and sebum production at puberty are stimulated by androgens. Growth hormone and thyroid hormones also affect sebum production.

Nails

A nail is a transparent plate of keratin derived from an invagination of epidermis on the dorsum of the terminal phalanx of a digit (Fig. 1.6). The nail plate is the product of cell division in the nail matrix, which lies deep to the proximal nail fold, but is partly visible as the pale 'half-moon' (lunula) at the base of the nail. The nail plate adheres firmly to the underlying nail bed. The cuticle is an extension of

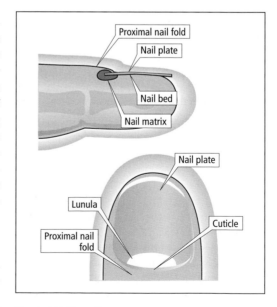

Figure 1.6 The nail.

the horny layer of the proximal nail fold onto the nail plate. It forms a seal between the nail plate and proximal nail fold, preventing penetration of extraneous material.

Nail growth is continuous throughout life, but is more rapid in youth than in old age. The average rate of growth of fingernails is approximately 1 mm per week, and the time taken for a fingernail to grow from matrix to free edge is about 6 months. Nails on the dominant hand grow slightly more rapidly than those on the non-dominant hand. Toenails grow at one-third the rate of fingernails, and take about 18 months to grow from matrix to free edge.

Many factors affect nail growth rate. It is increased in psoriasis, and may be speeded up in the presence of inflammatory change around the nail. A severe systemic upset can produce a sudden slowing of nail growth, causing a transverse groove in each nail plate. These grooves, known as Beau's lines, subsequently become visible as the nails grow out. Nail growth may also be considerably slowed in the digits of a limb immobilized in plaster.

The dermis

The dermis is a layer of connective tissue lying beneath the epidermis, and forms the bulk of the skin. The dermis and epidermis interdigitate via downward epidermal projections (rete ridges), and upward dermal projections (dermal papillae) (Figs 1.1 & 1.3). The main feature of the dermis is a network of interlacing fibres, mostly collagen, but with some elastin. These fibres give the dermis great strength and elasticity. The collagen and elastin fibres, which are protein, are embedded in a ground substance of mucopolysaccharides (glycosaminoglycans).

The main cellular elements of the dermis are fibroblasts, mast cells and macrophages. Fibroblasts synthesize the connective tissue matrix of the dermis, and are usually found in close proximity to collagen and elastin fibres. Mast cells are specialized secretory cells present throughout the dermis, but they are more numerous around blood vessels and appendages. They contain granules whose contents include mediators such as histamine, prostaglandins, leukotrienes, and eosinophil and neutrophil chemotactic factors. Macrophages are phagocytic cells that originate in the bone marrow, and they act as scavengers of cell debris and extracellular material. The dermis is also richly supplied with blood vessels, lymphatics, nerves and sensory receptors. Beneath the dermis, a layer of subcutaneous fat separates the skin from underlying fascia and muscle.

Dermatoglyphics

Fingerprints, the characteristic elevated ridge patterns on the fingertips of humans, are unique to each individual. The fingers and toes, and the palms and soles, are covered with a system of ridges which form patterns. The term 'dermatoglyphics' is applied to the configuration of the ridges. If you look closely at your hands you will see these tiny ridges, which are separate from the skin creases. On the tips of the fingers there are three basic patterns: arches, loops and whorls (Fig. 1.7). The loops are subdivided into ulnar or radial, depending on whether the loop is open to the ulnar or radial side of the hand. A triangular intersection of these ridges is known as a triradius, and these triradii are not only present on fingertips, but also at the base of each finger, and usually on the proximal part of the palm.

Not only are the ridge patterns of fingerprints useful for the identification and conviction of those who covet their neighbours' goods, but characteristic dermatoglyphic abnormalities frequently accompany many chromosomal aberrations.

Functions of the skin

Skin is like wax paper that holds everything in without dripping. (Art Linkletter, *A Child's Garden of Misinformation*, 1965)

It is obvious from the complex structure of the skin that it is not there simply to hold all the other bits of the body together. Some of the functions of skin are as follows:

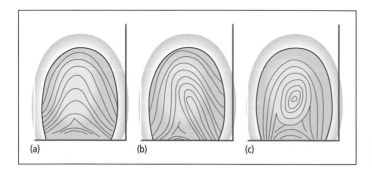

(a) (b) (c)

Figure 1.7 Dermatoglyphics: (a) arch; (b) loop; (c) whorl.

Skin functions

- Prevents loss of essential body fluids
- Protects against entry of toxic environmental chemicals and microorganisms
- Immunological functions
- Protects against damage from UV radiation
- Regulates body temperature
- Synthesis of vitamin D
- Important in sexual attraction and social interaction

In the absence of a stratum corneum, we would lose significant amounts of water to the environment, and rapidly become dehydrated. The stratum corneum, with its overlapping cells and intercellular lipid, blocks diffusion of water into the environment. If it is removed by stripping with tape, water loss to the environment increases 10-fold or more.

It is also quite an effective barrier to the penetration of external agents. However, this barrier capacity is considerably reduced if the stratum corneum is hydrated, or its lipid content is reduced by the use of lipid solvents. The structural integrity of the stratum corneum also protects against invasion by microorganisms and, when there is skin loss, for example in burns or toxic epidermal necrolysis, infection is a major problem. Other factors, such as the acid pH of sweat and sebaceous secretions, antimicrobial peptides (AMPs) known as *defensins* and *cathelicidins* that kill a variety of microbes, and complement components all contribute to antibacterial activity. The rarity of fungal infection of the scalp in adults is thought to be re-

lated to changes at puberty in the fatty acid composition of sebum, its constituents after puberty having fungistatic activity.

The skin is an immunologically competent organ and plays an important part in host defence against 'foreign' material. The dendritic Langerhans cells are antigen-presenting cells that take up antigens, process them and migrate to regional lymph nodes where the antigens, in association with major histocompatibility (MHC) class II, are presented to receptors on T cells. A naive T cell that interacts with an antigen proliferates to form a clone that will recognize the antigen if re-exposed to it. Such primed (memory) T cells circulate around the body. If the antigen is encountered again, the primed T cells are activated, and secrete cytokines that cause lymphocytes, polymorphonuclear leukocytes and monocytes to move into the area, thereby causing inflammation. This mechanism also forms the basis of the inflammatory reaction in allergic contact dermatitis.

Cytokines are polypeptides and glycoproteins secreted by cells (for example lymphocytes, macrophages and keratinocytes). They include interleukins, interferons (IFN), tumour necrosis factor (TNF), colony-stimulating factors and growth factors. Their main role is to regulate inflammatory and immune responses.

Although a detailed discussion of immunology and inflammation is beyond the scope of this book, it is important for you to understand some of the basic mechanisms involved for a variety of reasons, not least because such knowledge is necessary in order to comprehend the modes of action of the increasingly sophisticated treatments being developed. For example, biological therapies. 'Biologicals' are being used to treat psoriasis (Chapter 8) by targeting components of its pathomechanism, principally T cells and cytokines, with monoclonal antibodies that include efalizumab, which inhibits T-cell activation, and infliximab, which is an antibody to TNF-alpha (TNF-α).

The protective effect of melanin against UV damage has already been mentioned, but in addition to this there is an important system of enzymes responsible for repair of UV-damaged DNA. Such damage is occurring continuously, and the consequences of a non-functioning repair system can be seen in the recessively inherited disorder xeroderma pigmentosum (XP). In XP, cumulative UV damage leads to development of skin neoplasia in childhood.

The skin is a vital part of the body's temperature regulation system. The body core temperature is regulated by a temperature-sensitive area in the hypothalamus, and this is influenced by the temperature of the blood which perfuses it. The response of the skin to cold is vasoconstriction and a marked reduction in blood flow, decreasing transfer of heat to the body surface. The response to heat is vasodilatation, an increase in skin blood flow and loss of heat to the environment. Perspiration helps to cool the body by evaporation of sweat. These thermoregulatory functions are impaired in certain skin disease—patients suffering from exfoliative dermatitis (erythroderma) radiate heat to their environment because their skin blood flow is considerably increased and they are unable to control this by vasoconstriction. In a cold environment their central core temperature drops, in spite of producing metabolic heat by shivering, and they may die of hypothermia.

Vitamin D (cholecalciferol) is produced in the skin by the action of UV light on dehydrocholesterol. In those whose diets are deficient in vitamin D, this extra source of the vitamin can be important.

The skin is also a huge sensory receptor, perceiving heat, cold, pain, light touch and pressure, and even tickle. As you are probably still grappling with the conundrum of the biological significance of hairy ears in the elderly male, try switching your thoughts to the benefits of tickly armpits!

In addition to all these mechanistic functions, the skin plays an essential aesthetic role in social interaction and sexual attraction.

Hence, you can see that your skin is doing a good job. Apart from looking pleasant, it is saving you from becoming a cold, UV-damaged, brittle-boned, desiccated 'prune'.

Chapter 2

Approach to the diagnosis of dermatological disease

Baglivi has said, "The patient is the doctor's best text-book". That "text-book", however, has to be introduced to the student and those who effect the introductions are not always wise. (Dannie Abse, Doctors and Patients)

The dermatologist's art is giving a disease a long Greek name . . . and then a topical steroid. (Anon)

Diagnosis

- Provides a working label which will be recognized by others
- Implies some commonality with other patients with the same disease state or condition: in aetiology; pathology; clinical features; responsiveness to treatment
- Offers a prognosis and information about contagion or heredity
- Gives access to treatment modalities

Introduction

Dermatology is essentially a specialty where clinical information is at the forefront of the diagnostic process, and it is important for any aspiring clinician to realize that, before prescribing treatment or offering prognostic information about a patient's problem, he or she must first make a diagnosis. This chapter is about reaching a diagnosis in a patient with a skin disorder.

The value of a diagnosis

The facts on which a clinician makes a diagnosis *must* always come first and foremost from the patient, and there is no substitute for talking to and examining patients. This is especially true of skin disease.

A diagnosis is a short statement about a disease state or condition.

Dermatological diagnosis

That which we call a rose,
by any other name would smell as sweet
(Shakespeare, *Romeo and Juliet*)

Aspiring dermatologists must begin by becoming familiar with the diagnostic labels used in the description and classification of skin disease. This can seem daunting, but remember that diagnostic labels in medicine are bound by convention and rooted in history: the nomenclature of disease, and its signs and symptoms, has emerged from hundreds of years of classification and categorization. There is nothing special about dermatology, except perhaps in the degree to which subtle clinical variations are afforded separate names. The fact that diagnostic terms often bear no relationship to modern thinking is not of itself important. An apple is still an apple, even if we don't know who first called it that or why!

Therefore, as in any other branch of medicine, the diagnostic terminology in dermatology has to be learned. This is not as hard as it may at first seem. In the same way that someone moving to a foreign country has to become used to a new vocabulary, the dermatological tyro who pays attention rapidly becomes acquainted with the more common skin diseases (e.g. eczema, psoriasis or warts). In time, he or she will also begin to recognize rarer disorders and less 'classical' variants of more common ones. However, this remains a dynamic process which involves seeing, reading, asking and learning—always with the eyes, ears and mind open!

The steps to making a dermatological diagnosis

In principle, there is nothing difficult about dermatological diagnosis. The process of identifying skin diseases consists of taking a history, examining the patient, and performing investigations where necessary. In practice, many dermatologists will ask questions *after* a quick look to assess the problem, and also during the formal examination. However, we should consider the elements of the process separately.

A dermatological history contains most of the questions you will be used to asking: onset and duration, fluctuation, nature of symptoms, past history. There are some differences, however, which are largely in the emphasis placed on certain aspects, shown above:

There are also specific features of dermatological histories to watch out for.

Symptoms

Patients with skin disease talk about symptoms, especially itching, which you may not have met before. You will have to learn to assess and quantify these. You will soon get used to this. For example, a severe itch will keep patients awake or stop them from concentrating at work or school.

Patients' language

Be careful about terms that patients use to describe their skin problems. In Leicestershire, where the authors work, weals are often called 'blisters' and it is easy to be misled. Always ask the patient to describe precisely what he or she means by a specific term.

Quality of life

It may be helpful to assess the impact of the problem on the patient's normal daily activities and self-image: work, school, sleep, self-confidence, personal relationships.

Patient preconceptions

Patients often have their own ideas about the cause of skin problems and will readily offer them! For example, washing powder or detergent is almost

---

Dermatological history

Past history
Should include:
- General problems, such as diabetes and TB
- Past skin problems
- Significant allergies

Family history
- Some disorders are infectious; others have strong genetic backgrounds

Occupation and hobbies
- The skin is frequently affected by materials encountered at work and in the home

Therapy
- Not only *systemic* medication but also *topical*; many patients apply multiple creams and ointments; topicals may be medicinal (patients nearly always forget their names)

BUT
- *Topical medication* may also be self-administered as part of a 'cosmetic' regimen

---

universally considered to be a major cause of rashes, and injuries to be triggers of skin tumours. Never ignore what you are told, but take care to sieve the information in the light of your findings.

Watch out, too, for the very high expectations of many patients. They know that visible evidence is there for all to see: dermatology often truly requires a 'spot' diagnosis! Everyone from the patient and his/her relatives to the local greengrocer can see the problem and express their opinion.

Examination

The next step is to examine the patient. Wise counsels maintain that you should *always* examine a patient from head to foot. In reality this can be hard on both patient and doctor, especially if the problem is a solitary wart on the thumb! However, as a general rule, and especially with inflammatory dermatoses and conditions with several lesions, it is important to have an overall look at the sites involved. You may also find the unexpected, such as melanomas and other skin cancers.

Inspect *and palpate* the lesion(s) or rash (it may help to use a magnifying hand lens). The fundamental elements of a good dermatological examination are:

1 Site and/or distribution of the problem.
2 Characteristics of individual lesion(s).
3 Examination of 'secondary' sites.
4 'Special' techniques.

Unfortunately, names and terms can appear to get in the way of learning in dermatology. Indeed this seems to be one reason why many clinicians claim that dermatology is a mysterious and impenetrable mixture of mumbo-jumbo and strange potions. There is really no need for this attitude: the terms in use have developed for good reasons. They provide a degree of precision and a framework for diagnosis and decision making. Try to familiarize yourself with them, and to apply them correctly. They will provide the building-blocks with which you will go on to make dermatological diagnoses. So, in the early days, describe everything you see in these terms as far as possible.

Dermatological assessment

1 **Site(s) and/or distribution.** This can be very helpful: for example, psoriasis has a predilection for knees, elbows, scalp and lower back; eczema favours the flexures in children; acne occurs predominantly on the face and upper trunk; basal cell carcinomas are more common on the head and neck
2 **Characteristics of individual lesion(s):**
   • **The type.** Some simple preliminary reading is essential. Use Table 2.1 for the most common and important terms and their definitions
   • **The size.** Size is best *measured*, rather than being a comparison with peas, oranges or coins of the realm
   • **The shape.** Lesions may be various shapes, e.g. round, oval, annular, linear or 'irregular'; straight edges and angles may suggest external factors
   • **The outline and border.** The outline is irregular in a superficial spreading melanoma, but smooth in most benign lesions; the border is well defined in psoriasis, but blurred in most patches of eczema
   • **The colour.** It is always useful to note the colour: red, purple, brown, slate-black, etc.
   • **Surface features** (Table 2.1). It is helpful to assess whether the surface is smooth or rough, and to distinguish crust (dried serum) from scale (hyperkeratosis); some assessment of scale can be helpful, e.g. 'silvery' in psoriasis
   • **The texture—superficial? deep?** Use your fingertips on the surface; assess the depth and position in or beneath the skin; lift scale or crust to see what is underneath; try to make the lesion blanch with pressure
3 **Secondary sites.** Look for additional features which may assist in diagnosis. Good examples of this include:
   • The nails in psoriasis
   • The fingers and wrists in scabies
   • The toe-webs in fungal infections
   • The mouth in lichen planus
4 **'Special' techniques.** These will be covered in the appropriate chapters, but there are some tricks, e.g.
   • Scraping a psoriatic plaque for capillary bleeding
   • The Nikolsky sign in blistering diseases
   • 'Diascopy' in suspected cutaneous tuberculosis

It is fair to say that in inflammatory dermatoses a complication is having to decide *which lesion or lesions to select* for this descriptive process. Skin diseases are dynamic. Some lesions in any rash will be very early, some very late, and some at various intermediate evolutionary stages.

Table 2.1 Types and characteristics of lesions (Fig 2.1).

Lesion characteristics
• Macule: a flat, circumscribed area of skin discoloration
• Papule: a circumscribed elevation of the skin less than 0.5 cm in diameter
• Nodule: a circumscribed visible or palpable lump, larger than 0.5 cm
• Plaque: a circumscribed, disc-shaped, elevated area of skin:
'small' <2 cm in diameter
'large' >2 cm in diameter
• Vesicle: a small visible collection of fluid (<0.5 cm in diameter)
• Bulla: a large visible collection of fluid (>0.5 cm)
• Pustule: a visible accumulation of pus
• Ulcer: a loss of epidermis (often with loss of underlying dermis and subcutis as well)
• Weal: a circumscribed, elevated area of cutaneous oedema

Surface characteristics
• Scale: visible and palpable flakes due to aggregation and/or abnormalities of shed epidermal cells
• Crust: accumulated dried exudate, e.g. serum
• Horn: an elevated projection of keratin
• Excoriation: a secondary, superficial ulceration, due to scratching
• Maceration: an appearance of surface softening due to constant wetting
• Lichenification: a flat-topped thickening of the skin often secondary to scratching.

Try to examine as many patients as you can: frequent exposure to skin diseases helps you to develop an ability to recognize those lesions which provide the most useful diagnostic information.

This diagnostic process will gradually become one that you will perform increasingly easily and confidently as experience develops.

Investigation

Inevitably, history and examination alone will not always provide all the information required. There are some skin disorders in which further investigation is nearly always necessary: either to confirm a diagnosis with important prognostic or therapeutic implications (e.g. blistering disorders), or to seek an underlying, associated systemic disorder (e.g. in generalized pruritus). These situations are covered later in the appropriate chapters. The advances in modern genetics, too, mean that blood (or other tissues) can be analysed for evidence of specific defects. Sometimes clinical findings alone will not produce a satisfactory working diagnosis, or further information is required in order to plan optimal management.

A number of important techniques are available to provide further information. Some of these, such as appropriate blood tests and swabs for bacteriology and virology, should be familiar from other branches of medicine, and are fully covered in other introductory textbooks. Others, however, are more specific to dermatological investigation. Common, useful investigations in skin diseases include the following:

• Blood tests—for underlying systemic abnormalities and, increasingly, for genetic analysis.
• Swabs and other samples—for infections.
• Wood's light—some disorders/features are easier to see.
• Skin scrapes or nail clippings—microscopy and mycological culture.
• Skin biopsy—histopathology; electron microscopy; immunopathology; DNA phenotyping.
• Prick tests—occasionally helpful in elucidating type I allergies (they have little or no place in the investigation of eczema).
• Patch tests—for evidence of contact allergy.

Wood's light

This is a nickel oxide-filtered UV light source, used to highlight three features of skin disease:
1 Certain organisms which cause scalp ringworm produce green fluorescence (useful in initial diagnosis and helpful in assessing therapy).
2 The organism responsible for erythrasma fluoresces coral-pink.
3 Some pigmentary disorders are more clearly visible in this light—particularly the pale patches of tuberous sclerosis, and café-au-lait marks of neurofibromatosis.

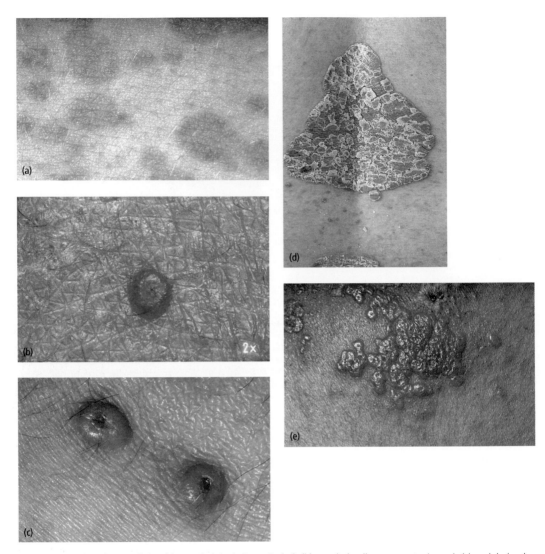

Figure 2.1 Lesion characteristics: (a) macule (pityriasis versicolor); (b) papule (molluscum contagiosum); (c) nodule (nodular prurigo); (d) plaque (psoriasis); (e) vesicle (herpes zoster); (f) bulla (bullous insect bite reaction); (g) pustule; (h) ulcer (venous ulcer); (i) weal (urticaria/dermographism).

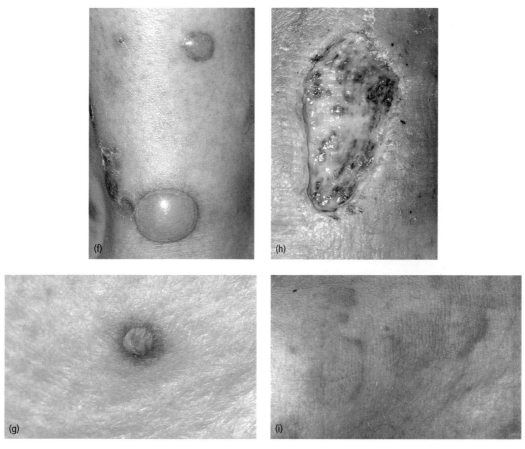

Figure 2.1 *Continued*

Wood's light can also be used to induce fluorescence in the urine in some of the porphyrias.

Scrapings/clippings

Material from the skin, hair or nails can be examined directly under the microscope and/or sent for culture. This is particularly useful in suspected fungal infection, or in a search for scabies mites (see Chapters 4 & 5). Scraping lightly at the epidermis will lift scales from the surface of the suspicious area.

The scales are placed on a microscope slide, covered with 10% potassium hydroxide (KOH) and a coverslip. After a few minutes to dissolve some of the epidermal cell membranes, they can be examined. It is helpful to add some Parker Quink ink if an infection with *Malassezia* (*Pityrosporum*) (the cause of pityriasis versicolor) is suspected. Nail clippings can also be treated this way, but need stronger solutions of KOH, or longer to dissolve.

Microscopy of hair may also provide information about fungal infections, may reveal structural hair shaft abnormalities in certain genetic disorders and can be useful in distinguishing some causes of excessive hair loss (see Chapter 13).

Scrape/smear preparations are also used as a diagnostic aid by some dermatologists for the cytodiagnosis of suspected viral blisters and pemphigus, using a 'Tzanck preparation', which enables material to be examined directly in the clinic.

Skin biopsy

Skin biopsy is a very important technique in the diagnosis of many skin disorders. In some, it is critical to have confirmation of a clinical diagnosis before embarking on treatment. Good examples of this are skin cancers, bullous disorders, and infections such as tuberculosis and leprosy. In others it is necessary to take a biopsy because clinical information alone has not provided all the answers.

There are two methods commonly used to obtain a skin sample for laboratory examination:
1 Incisional/excisional biopsy.
2 Punch biopsy.

Specimens obtained by either technique may be sent for conventional histopathology—normally fixed immediately in formol-saline—and/or other specialized examinations, for example for DNA phenotyping of specific cells or for viral DNA. For immunopathology the skin is usually snap frozen, but for electron microscopy skin is best fixed in glutaraldehyde.

Always check the details with the laboratory before you start.

Incisional/excisional biopsy

This provides good-sized samples (which can be divided for different purposes if required) and can be

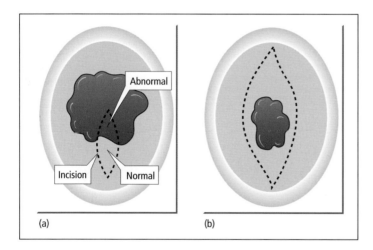

Figure 2.2 The technique for incisional (a) and (b) excisional biopsy.

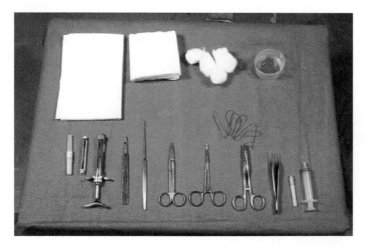

Figure 2.3 Equipment needed for an incisional/excisional biopsy: sterile towel; gauze squares; cotton-wool balls; galley pot containing antiseptic; needle; cartridge of lidocaine (lignocaine) and dental syringe; scalpel; skin hook; scissors; small artery forceps; needle holder and suture; fine, toothed forceps; needle and syringe (alternative to dental syringe).

used to remove quite large lesions (see Figs 2.2 & 2.3).

1 Administer local anaesthetic. 1–2% lidocaine (lignocaine) is usual; addition of 1 : 10000 adrenaline (epinephrine) helps reduce bleeding, but **never** use on fingers and toes.

2 For incisional (diagnostic) biopsy. Make two cuts forming an ellipse; ensure that the specimen is taken across the edge of the lesion, retaining a margin of normal perilesional skin (Fig. 2.2a).

3 For complete excision. Widen the ellipse around the whole lesion (Fig. 2.2b); ensure that the excision edge is cut vertically and *does not* slant in towards the tumour, which can result in inadequate deeper excision (Fig. 2.4).

4 Repair the defect. Edges left by either incisional or excisional biopsy are brought neatly together with sutures; the choice of suture material is not critical, but for the best cosmetic result use the finest possible, preferably a synthetic monofilament suture (e.g. prolene).

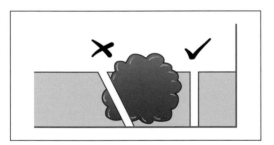

Figure 2.4 Excisional biopsy: the correct (✓) and incorrect (✗) excision edge.

Note: if there will be significant tension on the suture line, consider asking a trained plastic or dermatological surgeon for advice.

Punch biopsy

This is much quicker, but produces small samples and is only appropriate for diagnostic biopsies or removing tiny lesions (see Fig. 2.5a–c):

1 Administer local anaesthesia (see above).

2 Push the punch biopsy blade into the lesion using a circular motion.

3 Lift out the small plug, and separate with scissors or a scalpel blade.

4 Achieve haemostasis with silver nitrate or a small suture.

Patch tests

If a contact allergic dermatitis is suspected, a patch test is performed. In this process possible allergens are usually diluted in suitable vehicles. The test materials are placed in small discs in contact with the skin (usually on the back) for 48 h (Fig. 2.6a). A positive reaction (at 48 h, or occasionally later) confirms a delayed hypersensitivity (type IV) reaction to the offending substance (Fig. 2.6b).

This technique can be extended to include testing for photoallergy.

Conclusion

You are now ready to start examining and talking to patients with skin disease. Attend some dermatology clinics and put these principles into

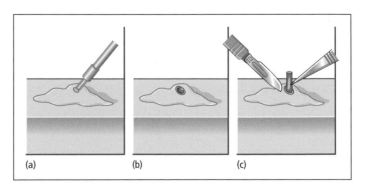

Figure 2.5 (a–c) The technique for a punch biopsy.

(a) (b) (c)

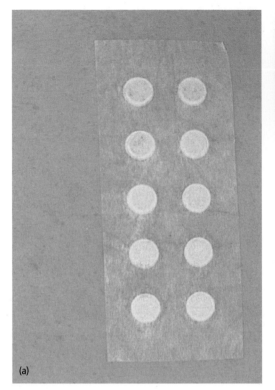
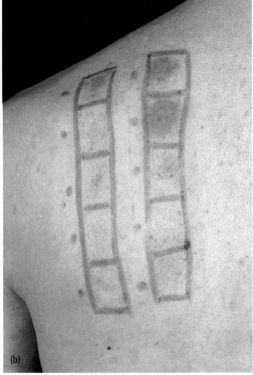

Figure 2.6 Patch testing: (a) metal cups containing allergens; (b) positive patch test reactions.

practice. When seeing patients, try to retain a mental picture of their skin lesions. Ask the dermatologist in charge what the diagnosis is in each instance, and make sure that you read a little about each entity when the clinic is over.

The remaining chapters of this book are designed to help you to make specific diagnoses, to provide your patients with information about their problems and to assist you in choosing appropriate treatment.

Chapter 3

Bacterial and viral infections

A mighty creature is the germ
Though smaller than the pachyderm
His customary dwelling place
Is deep within the human race
His childish pride he often pleases
By giving people strange diseases
Do you, my poppet, feel infirm?
You probably contain a germ
(Ogden Nash, *The Germ*)

Bacterial infections

Streptococcal infection

Cellulitis

Cellulitis is a bacterial infection of subcutaneous tissues that, in immunologically normal individuals, is usually caused by *Streptococcus pyogenes*. 'Erysipelas' is a term applied to superficial streptococcal cellulitis that has a well-demarcated edge. Occasionally, other bacteria are implicated in cellulitis—*Haemophilus influenzae* is an important cause of facial cellulitis in children, often in association with ipsilateral otitis media. In immunocompromised individuals, a variety of bacteria may be responsible for cellulitis.

Cellulitis frequently occurs on the legs, but other parts of the body may be affected—the face is a common site for erysipelas. The organisms may gain entry into the skin via minor abrasions, or fissures between the toes associated with tinea pedis, and leg ulcers provide a portal of entry in many cases. A frequent predisposing factor is oedema of the legs, and cellulitis is a common condition in elderly people, who often suffer from leg oedema of cardiac, venous or lymphatic origin.

The affected area becomes red, hot and swollen (Fig. 3.1), and blister formation and areas of skin necrosis may occur. The patient is pyrexial and feels unwell. Rigors may occur and, in elderly people, a toxic confusional state.

In presumed streptococcal cellulitis, penicillin is the treatment of choice, initially given as benzylpenicillin intravenously. If the leg is affected, bed rest is an important aspect of treatment. Where there is extensive tissue necrosis, surgical debridement may be necessary.

A particularly severe, deep form of cellulitis, involving fascia and muscles, is known as 'necrotizing fasciitis'. This disorder achieved notoriety a few years ago when it attracted the attention of the UK popular press and was described as being caused by a 'flesh-eating virus'. It is associated with extensive tissue necrosis and severe toxaemia, and is rapidly fatal unless urgent treatment, including excision of the affected area, is undertaken.

Some patients have recurrent episodes of cellulitis, each episode damaging lymphatics and leading to further oedema. These cases should be treated with prophylactic oral phenoxymethylpenicillin

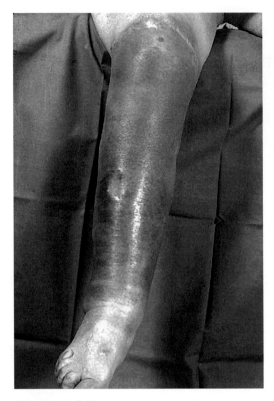

Figure 3.1 Cellulitis.

(penicillin V) or erythromycin, to prevent further episodes.

Staphylococcal infection

Folliculitis

Infection of the superficial part of a hair follicle with *Staphylococcus aureus* produces a small pustule on an erythematous base, centred on the follicle.

Mild folliculitis can be treated with a topical antibacterial agent, but if it is extensive a systemic antibiotic may be required.

Furunculosis ('boils')

A boil (furuncle) is the result of deep infection of a hair follicle by *S. aureus*. A painful abscess develops at the site of infection, and over a period of a few days becomes fluctuant and 'points' as a central pustule. Once the necrotic central core has been discharged, the lesion gradually resolves. In some patients, boils are a recurrent problem, but this is rarely associated with a significant underlying disorder. Such individuals may be nasal or perineal carriers of staphylococci, and organisms are transferred on the digits to various parts of the body.

Patients suffering from recurrent boils should have swabs taken from the nose for culture, and if found to be carrying staphylococci should be treated with a topical antibacterial such as mupirocin, applied to the nostrils. They may also be helped by an antibacterial bath additive, for example 2% triclosan, and a prolonged course of flucloxacillin.

Carbuncle

A carbuncle is a deep infection of a group of adjacent hair follicles with *S. aureus*. A frequent site for a carbuncle is the nape of the neck. Initially, the lesion is a dome-shaped area of tender erythema, but after a few days suppuration begins, and pus is discharged from multiple follicular orifices. Carbuncles are usually encountered in middle-aged and elderly men, and are associated with diabetes and debility. They are uncommon nowadays. Flucloxacillin should be given for treatment.

Impetigo

This is a contagious superficial infection which occurs in two clinical forms, non-bullous and bullous. Non-bullous impetigo is caused by *S. aureus*, streptococci or both organisms together. The streptococcal form predominates in warm, humid climates, for example the southern USA. Bullous impetigo is caused by *S. aureus*. Lesions may occur anywhere on the body. In the non-bullous form, the initial lesion is a small pustule which ruptures to leave an extending area of exudation and crusting (Fig. 3.2). The crusts eventually separate to leave areas of erythema, which fade without scarring. In the bullous form, large, superficial blisters develop. When these rupture, there is exudation and crusting, and the stratum corneum peels back at the edges of the lesions.

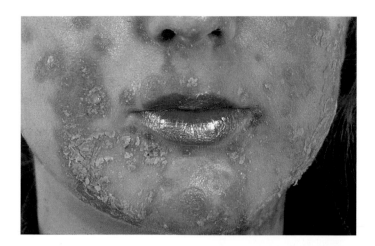

Figure 3.2 Impetigo.

Streptococcal impetigo may be associated with poststreptococcal acute glomerulonephritis.

Impetigo may occur as a secondary phenomenon in atopic eczema, scabies and head louse infection.

In localized infection, treatment with a topical antibiotic such as mupirocin will suffice, but, in more extensive infection, treatment with a systemic antibiotic such as flucloxacillin or erythromycin is indicated.

Staphylococcal scalded skin syndrome

This uncommon condition occurs as a result of infection with certain staphylococcal phage types that produce a toxin which splits the epidermis at the level of the granular layer. The superficial epidermis peels off in sheets, producing an appearance resembling scalded skin. Infants and young children are usually affected. It responds to parenteral therapy with flucloxacillin.

Erythrasma

Caused by a Gram-positive organism, *Corynebacterium minutissimum*, erythrasma occurs in intertriginous areas—axillae, groins and submammary regions. However, the most common site colonized by this organism is the toe-web spaces, where it produces a macerated scaling appearance identical to that caused by fungal infection. In other

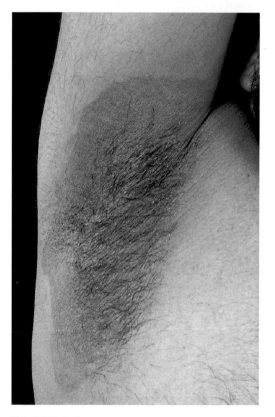

Figure 3.3 Erythrasma.

sites, it produces marginated brown areas with a fine, branny surface scale (Fig. 3.3). It is usually asymptomatic. *Corynebacterium minutissimum* produces a porphyrin that fluoresces a striking coral-pink under Wood's light.

Erythrasma may be treated with topical imidazoles (e.g. clotrimazole, miconazole), topical fusidic acid or a 2-week course of oral erythromycin.

Mycobacterial infection

Cutaneous tuberculosis

Cutaneous tuberculosis is now uncommon in Europe and the USA, but may be encountered in immigrants from other parts of the world where tuberculosis remains problematic.

Scrofuloderma

Scrofuloderma results from involvement of the skin overlying a tuberculous focus, usually a lymph node, most commonly in the neck. The clinical appearance is of multiple fistulae and dense scar tissue.

Lupus vulgaris

The majority of lesions of lupus vulgaris occur on the head and neck. The typical appearance is of a reddish-brown, nodular plaque (Fig. 3.4). When pressed with a glass slide (diascopy), the brown nodules, which are referred to as 'apple jelly' nodules, are more easily seen. The natural course is gradual peripheral extension, and in many cases this is extremely slow, over a period of years. Lupus vulgaris is a destructive process, and the cartilage of the nose and ears may be severely damaged.

Histology shows tubercles composed of epithelioid cells and Langhans giant cells, usually without central caseation. Tubercle bacilli are sparse. The tuberculin test is strongly positive. The patient should be investigated for an underlying focus of tuberculosis in other organs, but this is only found in a small proportion of cases.

Treatment should be with standard antituberculous chemotherapy.

There is a risk of the development of squamous cell carcinoma in the scar tissue of longstanding lupus vulgaris.

Warty tuberculosis

This occurs as a result of direct inoculation of tubercle bacilli into the skin of someone previously infected, who has a high degree of immunity. It may develop on the buttocks and thighs as a result of sitting on ground contaminated by infected sputum. The clinical appearance is of a warty plaque. It responds to standard antituberculous chemotherapy.

Tuberculides

This term is applied to skin lesions that occur in response to tuberculosis elsewhere in the body. They

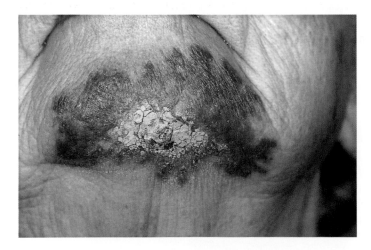

Figure 3.4 Lupus vulgaris on the chin.

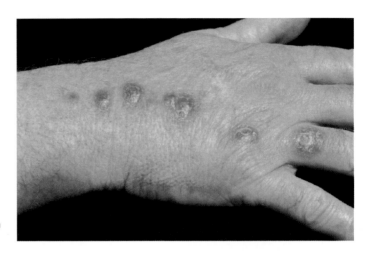

Figure **3.5** Fish tank granuloma showing sporotrichoid spread.

are probably the result of haematogenous dissemination of bacilli in individuals with a moderate or high degree of immunity. Included in this group are erythema induratum (Bazin's disease), papulonecrotic tuberculide and lichen scrofulosorum.

Atypical mycobacteria

The most common of the skin lesions produced by atypical mycobacteria is 'swimming pool' or 'fish tank' granuloma. This is usually a solitary granulomatous nodule, caused by inoculation of *Mycobacterium marinum* into the skin via an abrasion sustained whilst swimming, or (in tropical fish fanciers) whilst cleaning out the aquarium—often after the demise of the fish contained therein. Occasionally, in addition to the initial lesion, there are several secondary lesions in a linear distribution along the lines of lymphatics (sporotrichoid spread—because it resembles sporotrichosis) (Fig. 3.5). Most cases respond to treatment with minocycline.

Leprosy (Hansen's disease)

The Norwegian Armauer Hansen discovered the leprosy bacillus, *Mycobacterium leprae*, in 1873 and, if the possibility of leprosy enters into the discussion of differential diagnosis in the clinic, the eponymous title of this condition should always be used, because the fear of leprosy is so ingrained, even in countries where it is not endemic.

Leprosy has a wide distribution throughout the world, with most cases occurring in the tropics and subtropics, but population movements mean that the disease may be encountered anywhere in the world.

Leprosy is a disease of peripheral nerves, but it also affects the skin, and sometimes other tissues such as the eyes, the mucosa of the upper respiratory tract, the bones and the testes. Although it is infectious, the degree of infectivity is low. The incubation period is lengthy, probably several years, and it is likely that most patients acquire the infection in childhood. A low incidence of conjugal leprosy (leprosy acquired from an infected spouse) suggests that adults are relatively non-susceptible. The disease is acquired as a result of close physical contact with an infected person, the risk being much greater for contacts of lepromatous cases—the nasal discharges of these individuals are the main source of infection in the community.

The clinical pattern of disease is determined by the host's cell-mediated immune response to the organism. When this is well developed, tuberculoid leprosy occurs, in which skin and peripheral nerves are affected. Skin lesions are single, or few in number, and are well defined. They are macules or plaques that are hypopigmented in dark skin. The lesions are anaesthetic, sweating is absent, and hairs are reduced in number. Thickened branches of cutaneous sensory nerves may be palpable in the region of these lesions, and large peripheral nerves may also be palpable. The lepromin test is strongly positive. Histology shows well-defined tuberculoid granulomas, and bacilli are not seen. The Wade–Fite stain is used to demonstrate leprosy bacilli.

When the cell-mediated immune response is poor, the bacilli multiply unchecked and the patient develops lepromatous leprosy. The bacilli spread to involve not only the skin, but also the mucosa of the respiratory tract, the eyes, testes and bones. Skin lesions are multiple and nodular. The lepromin test is negative. Histology shows a diffuse granuloma throughout the dermis, and bacilli are present in large numbers.

In between these two extreme, 'polar' forms of leprosy is a spectrum of disease referred to as borderline leprosy, the clinical and histological features of which reflect different degrees of cell-mediated response to the bacilli. There is no absolute diagnostic test for leprosy—the diagnosis is based on clinical and histological features.

Tuberculoid leprosy is usually treated with a combination of dapsone and rifampicin for 6 months; lepromatous leprosy with dapsone, rifampicin and clofazimine for at least 24 months. The treatment of leprosy may be complicated by immunologically mediated 'reactional states', and should be supervised by someone experienced in leprosy management.

The leprosy spectrum

Tuberculoid
- One or two skin lesions only
- Good cell-mediated immune response
- Positive lepromin test
- Few bacilli

Borderline
- Scattered skin lesions
- Intermediate cell-mediated immune response
- Some organisms

Lepromatous
- Extensive skin lesions and involvement of other organs
- Poor cell-mediated immune response
- Negative lepromin test
- Numerous organisms

Viral infections

Warts

'Mr Lely, I desire you would use all your skill to paint my picture truly like me, and not flatter me at all; but remark all these roughnesses, pimples, warts, and everything as you see me, otherwise I will never pay a farthing for it'. (Oliver Cromwell to the artist Sir Peter Lely—origin of 'Warts and all')

Warts are benign epidermal neoplasms caused by viruses of the human papillomavirus (HPV) group. There are a number of different strains of HPV that produce different clinical types of warts. Warts are also known as 'verrucae', although the term verruca in popular usage is usually reserved for the plantar wart.

Common warts

These are raised, cauliflower-like lesions that occur most frequently on the hands (Fig. 3.6). They are extremely common in childhood and early adult life. They may be scattered, grouped or periungual in distribution. Common warts in children usually resolve spontaneously.

Common warts are usually treated with wart paints or cryotherapy. Preparations containing salicylic acid are often quite effective, and a wart paint should certainly be used for at least 3 months before considering alternative treatment.

Cryotherapy with liquid nitrogen can be used on warts that do not respond to wart paints. A simple applicator of cotton wool wrapped around the end of an orange stick may be used. This is dipped in the liquid nitrogen and then applied to the wart until it and a narrow rim of surrounding skin are frozen. Alternatively, a liquid nitrogen cryospray may be used. This is a painful procedure, and should not be inflicted on children—however, most tiny tots will, sensibly, retreat under the desk protesting loudly at first sight of the nitrogen evaporating in its container. Multiple warts usually require more than one application, and the optimum interval between treatments is 2–3 weeks.

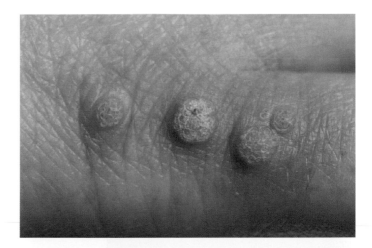

Figure 3.6 Viral warts.

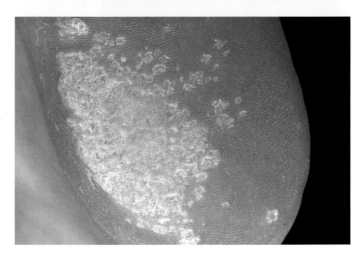

Figure 3.7 Mosaic plantar warts.

Plantar warts

Plantar warts may be solitary, scattered over the sole of the foot, or grouped together producing so-called 'mosaic' warts (Fig. 3.7). The typical appearance is of a small area of thickened skin which, when pared away, reveals numerous small black dots produced by thrombosed capillaries. Plantar warts are frequently painful. They must be distinguished from calluses and corns, which develop in areas of friction over bony prominences. Calluses are patches of uniformly thickened skin, and corns have a painful central plug of keratin that does not contain capillaries.

Treatment is with wart paints or cryotherapy, after paring down overlying keratin.

Plane warts

These are tiny, flat-topped, flesh-coloured warts which usually occur on the dorsa of the hands and the face (Fig. 3.8). They often occur in lines due to inoculation of the virus into scratches and abrasions. Plane warts are extremely difficult to treat effectively, and attempts at treatment may do more harm than good. They will resolve spontaneously eventually, and are best left alone.

Genital warts (condylomata acuminata)

In recent years, the importance of certain types of genital wart viruses in the aetiology of penile and cervical cancer has been recognized, and this has

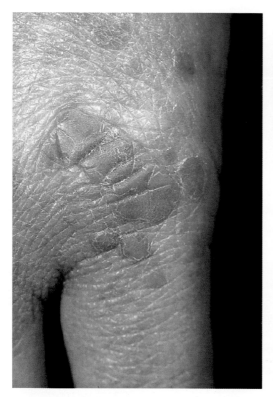

Figure 3.8 Plane warts.

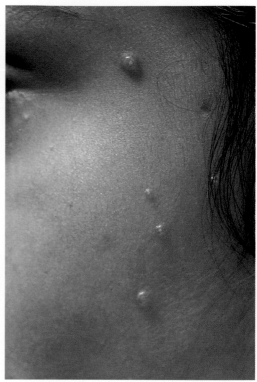

Figure 3.9 Molluscum contagiosum.

modified attitudes to what was previously considered a minor sexually transmitted inconvenience. It is now more appropriate that patients suffering from genital warts are seen and treated in a department of genitourinary medicine, so that coexisting sexually transmitted disease may be detected and treated, and sexual contacts traced and examined.

Molluscum contagiosum

The lesions of molluscum contagiosum are caused by a poxvirus. They are typically pearly, pink papules with a central umbilication filled with a keratin plug (Fig. 3.9). The lesions may occur anywhere on the body, but are most common on the head and neck area and the trunk. They are frequently grouped, and may be surrounded by a mild eczematous reaction. They may be very extensive in children with atopic eczema.

These lesions resolve spontaneously, and in infants and small children are best left alone to do so.

However, if parents of small children are anxious, they can be advised to squeeze each lesion between the thumbnails to express the central plug—this will often speed their resolution. In older children and adults, molluscum contagiosum can be treated by cryotherapy.

Orf

Orf is caused by a parapoxvirus. It is a disease of sheep that can be transmitted to humans. Those usually affected are people who bottle-feed lambs, and butchers and abattoir workers who handle the carcasses of sheep. The typical clinical picture is of a solitary, inflammatory papule that rapidly develops into a nodule of granulation tissue—usually on a finger, but occasionally on the face. The diagnosis can be confirmed by electron microscopy of smears from the granulation tissue. Orf lesions resolve spontaneously in 6–8 weeks, but the disease may act as a trigger for erythema multiforme.

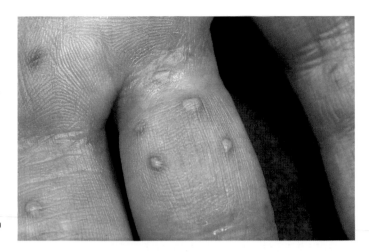

Figure 3.10 Hand, foot and mouth disease: vesicles on the hand.

Hand, foot and mouth disease

This is not related to foot and mouth disease of sheep and cattle, but is a harmless disease caused by Coxsackie virus infection, usually type A16. Characteristic small grey vesicles with a halo of erythema occur on the hands and feet (Fig. 3.10), and the buccal mucosa is studded with erosions resembling aphthous ulcers. The condition resolves within 2 weeks, and no treatment is required.

Herpes simplex

Herpes simplex is caused by herpes virus hominis (HSV). There are two antigenic types: type 1 is classically associated with the common 'cold sore' on the lips and face, and type 2 with genital herpes. However, neither has rigid territorial demarcation, and lesions anywhere may be caused by either antigenic type.

Primary herpes simplex

Initial contact with type 1 HSV usually occurs in early childhood, for example adults with cold sores kissing children, and any lesions that develop are often so mild that they are not noticed. Occasionally, however, a severe primary herpetic gingivostomatitis occurs, with painful erosions on the buccal mucosa and lips. Primary cutaneous herpes simplex may also occur, and in atopic eczema this can be very extensive and may be life-threatening (see eczema herpeticum below). Genital herpes may result from sexual transmission of type 2 HSV or orogenital transmission of type 1 HSV.

Physical contact during sport provides another means of HSV transmission—in rugby, herpes simplex thus acquired is known as 'scrumpox', and in wrestling as 'herpes gladiatorum'.

Following a primary infection, the virus settles in sensory ganglia, and may be triggered to produce recurrent lesions by a variety of stimuli. In immunodeficient individuals, for example those who are immunosuppressed following organ transplantation, or in association with human immunodeficiency virus (HIV) infection, herpes simplex infection may be clinically atypical and run a prolonged course.

Recurrent herpes simplex

Recurrent cold sores on the lips (herpes labialis) are common. Itching and discomfort in the affected area precedes, by a few hours, the eruption of a group of small vesicles. The vesicle contents subsequently become cloudy, and then crusting occurs, before resolution in about 10 days. The trigger for these episodes is often fever, but exposure to strong sunlight, and menstruation are also recognized precipitants. Occasionally, as a result of inoculation of the virus into a finger, painful episodes of 'herpetic whitlow' occur. The frequency of episodes of herpes simplex usually gradually declines with advancing age.

Labial herpes simplex is usually a minor cosmetic inconvenience, and does not require treatment. However, if episodes are frequent and troublesome, topical aciclovir may be of benefit. This blocks viral replication—it is not viricidal, and is not curative.

Herpes simplex and erythema multiforme

Recurrent herpes simplex can trigger erythema multiforme. Prophylactic oral aciclovir may be of considerable benefit in the management of severe cases.

Eczema herpeticum (Kaposi's varicelliform eruption)

This is a widespread herpes simplex infection that occurs in atopic eczema. The head and neck are frequently affected (Fig. 3.11), but lesions may spread rapidly to involve extensive areas of skin. Lymphadenopathy and constitutional upset may occur. If the disease is limited in distribution and the patient is seen early in its course, oral aciclovir therapy is appropriate. However, if the lesions are extensive, and the patient is unwell, they should be admitted to hospital and treated with intravenous aciclovir. If the patient is using topical steroid therapy to treat the eczema, this should be

stopped until the herpes has resolved. Eczema herpeticum may recur, but in many cases subsequent episodes tend to be less severe.

Herpes zoster (shingles)

Chickenpox and herpes zoster are both caused by the varicella-zoster virus. 'Shingles' is a distortion of the Latin *cingulum*, meaning a girdle.

Following an attack of chickenpox, the virus remains dormant in dorsal root ganglia until some stimulus reactivates it and causes shingles. Middle aged and elderly people are most often affected, but it occasionally occurs in childhood. It is also more frequent in immunosuppressed individuals.

Shingles usually affects a single dermatome, most commonly on the thorax or abdomen. The eruption may be preceded by pain in the region of the dermatome, and this occasionally leads to an incorrect diagnosis of internal pathology. The lesions consist of a unilateral band of grouped vesicles on an erythematous base (Fig. 3.12). The contents of the vesicles are initially clear, but subsequently become cloudy. There may be scattered outlying vesicles on the rest of the body, and these tend to be more numerous in elderly people. However, numerous outlying vesicles (disseminated zoster) are also seen in immunosuppressed individuals, and their presence should prompt further investigation of the patient. After a few days, the vesicles dry up and form crusts, and in most cases

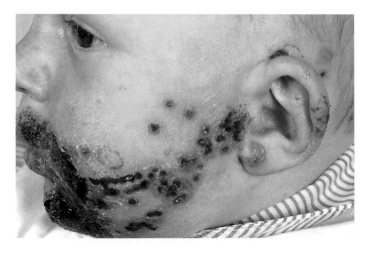

Figure 3.11 Eczema herpeticum.

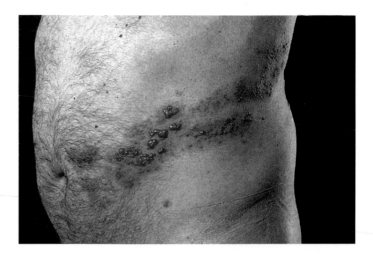

Figure 3.12 Herpes zoster.

the eruption resolves within 2 weeks. In elderly people, shingles can produce quite severe erosive changes that take considerably longer to heal. Even in milder cases there is usually some residual scarring.

The most troublesome aspect of shingles is the persistence of pain after the lesions have healed (postherpetic neuralgia). This may be severe, and is particularly distressing for elderly patients.

Sacral zoster

Involvement of the sacral segments may cause acute retention of urine in association with the rash.

Trigeminal zoster

Herpes zoster may affect any of the divisions of the trigeminal nerve, but the ophthalmic division is the most frequently involved (Fig. 3.13). Ocular problems such as conjunctivitis, keratitis and/or iridocyclitis may occur if the nasociliary branch of the ophthalmic division is affected (indicated by vesicles on the side of the nose), and patients with ophthalmic zoster should be examined by an ophthalmologist.

Involvement of the maxillary division of the trigeminal nerve produces vesicles on the cheek, and unilateral vesicles on the palate.

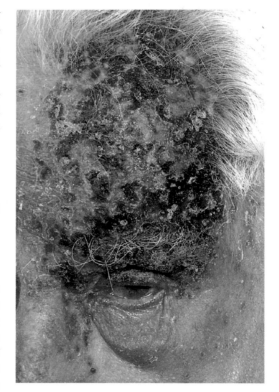

Figure 3.13 Ophthalmic zoster.

Motor zoster

Occasionally, in addition to skin lesions in a sensory dermatome, motor fibres are affected, leading to muscle weakness.

Treatment of herpes zoster

Many cases do not require any treatment. However, in severe cases, oral aciclovir, valaciclovir or famciclovir are of benefit. In disseminated zoster in immunosuppressed patients, intravenous aciclovir can be life saving.

Pain relief is often difficult to achieve in postherpetic neuralgia, and patients with severe discomfort should be referred to a pain relief specialist.

Chapter 4

Fungal infections

Introduction

The fungi that may cause human disease include the dermatophytes (Greek, meaning 'skin plants') and the yeast-like fungus *Candida albicans*, which are responsible for superficial fungal infections confined to the skin, hair and nails, and mucous membranes. Other fungi can invade living tissue to cause deep infections, which may remain localized (mycetoma) or cause systemic disease (e.g. histoplasmosis).

The dermatophytes are a group of fungi that are responsible for so-called 'ringworm' infections. The vegetative phase of dermatophyte fungi consists of septate hyphae which form a branching network (mycelium). *Candida albicans* is an organism composed of round or oval cells which divide by budding. Apart from its yeast form, it may produce pseudohyphae consisting of numerous cells in a linear arrangement or, in certain circumstances, true septate hyphae.

Dermatophyte infections

It is very easy to become totally confused by the terminology employed in fungal infection, and end up not knowing your tinea cruris from your *Trichophyton rubrum*. Hence, a novice is best advised to stick to simple terminology. The term 'ringworm', followed by 'of the feet, of the groin, of the scalp', etc., is a simple way of indicating the location of the infection. If you feel in more classical mood you may use 'tinea' (Latin, meaning 'a gnawing worm') followed by 'pedis', 'cruris', 'capitis', etc.

The dermatophyte fungi are named according to their genus (*Microsporum*, *Trichophyton* or *Epidermophyton*) and their species (e.g. *M. canis*, *T. rubrum*), and they can be distinguished from one another in culture. An experienced dermatologist may be able to suggest that a certain fungus is responsible for a particular case of ringworm, but the only way to establish its identity precisely is by culture.

Some fungi are confined to humans (anthropophilic), others principally affect animals (zoophilic) but occasionally infect humans. When animal fungi cause human skin lesions their presence often provokes a severe inflammatory reaction (e.g. cattle ringworm). Dermatophytes grow only in keratin—the stratum corneum of the skin, hair and nails. Infection is usually acquired by contact with keratin debris carrying fungal hyphae—for example, the lady who developed ringworm on the buttocks as a result of her husband's habit of cutting his toenails with his feet resting on the lavatory seat.

Tinea pedis (athlete's foot)

This is the most common of the dermatophyte infections, and usually presents as scaling, itchy areas in the toe-webs, particularly between the third and fourth, and fourth and fifth toes, or on

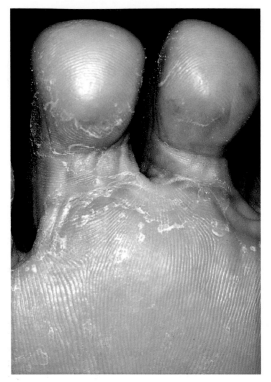

Figure 4.1 Athlete's foot.

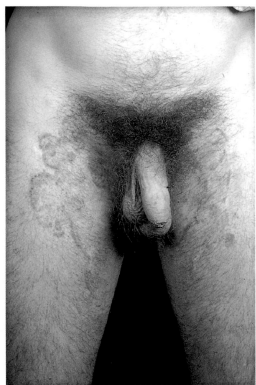

Figure 4.2 Tinea cruris.

the soles (Fig. 4.1). It is usually acquired from contact with infected keratin debris on the floors of swimming pools and showers. Sometimes there is extensive involvement of the soles and sides of the feet (so-called moccasin tinea pedis, because of its similarity to the shape of that soft leather shoe). The condition may also spread on to the dorsa of the feet. Occasionally, athlete's foot follows a pattern of episodic vesiculobullous lesions on the soles, occurring particularly during warm weather. The feet are frequently asymmetrically involved in fungal infection, in contrast with eczema, in which the involvement is usually symmetrical.

Tinea cruris

This is common in men and rare in women. The clinical picture is characteristic, and should be easy to distinguish from intertrigo, flexural psoriasis and flexural seborrhoeic dermatitis. A scaly, erythematous margin gradually spreads down the medial aspects of the thighs (Fig. 4.2), and may extend backwards to involve the perineum and buttocks. The source of the infection is nearly always the patient's feet, so they should be examined for evidence of athlete's foot or fungal nail dystrophy. The fungus is presumably transferred to the groins on fingers that have scratched itchy feet and then scratched groins, or on towels.

Tinea corporis

Tinea on the body typically has an inflammatory edge with central clearing (Fig. 4.3), but it is relatively uncommon. The differential diagnosis includes granuloma annulare and erythema annulare. In the former, there is a raised margin, but no scaling. The latter provides more diagnostic difficulty because the inflammatory margin is scaly. If fungal infection is suspected, scrapings should be

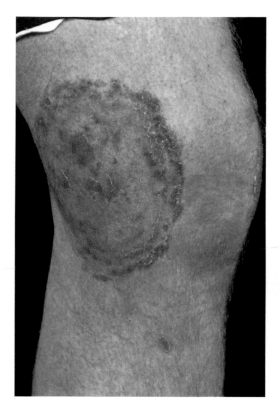

Figure 4.3 Tinea corporis.

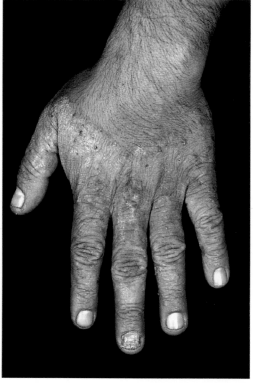

Figure 4.4 Tinea on the dorsum of the hand. Note involvement of middle finger nail.

examined microscopically for hyphae. In adults, the source of the fungus is usually the feet, whereas in children it has usually spread from the scalp.

Tinea manuum

Ringworm on the hand is usually unilateral. On the palm, the appearance is of mild scaling erythema, whereas on the dorsum there is more obvious inflammatory change, with a well-defined edge (Fig. 4.4). The source of the fungus is almost invariably the patient's feet.

Tinea unguium

Toenail fungal dystrophy is very common in adults, and is invariably associated with athlete's foot. The involvement usually starts laterally as yellowish streaks in the nail plate (Fig. 4.5), but gradually the whole nail becomes thickened, discoloured and friable. *Trichophyton rubrum* is usually

the cause. The great toenails are often the first to be affected, and pressure from footwear on the thickened nails may produce considerable discomfort.

A less common pattern is white superficial onychomycosis, in which the dorsal part of the nail plate shows white patches, and *T. mentagrophytes* is usually responsible for this.

Rapid proximal invasion of the nail plate, producing white discolouration, is a pattern seen in AIDS patients.

Fingernails are less commonly affected. The changes in the nail plate are similar to those seen in toenails (Fig. 4.6).

Tinea capitis

Tinea capitis is principally a disease of childhood, and is rare in adults. This is thought to be related to a change in the fatty acid constituents of sebum

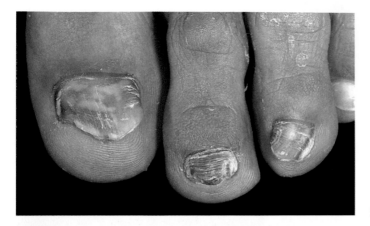

Figure 4.5 Tinea of the toenails.

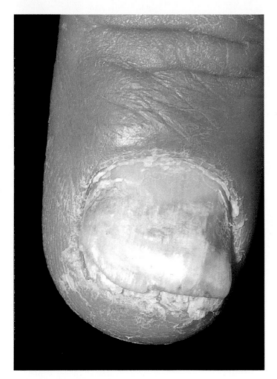

Figure 4.6 Tinea of a fingernail.

around the time of puberty. Postpubertal sebum contains fungistatic fatty acids. The principal fungi responsible for scalp ringworm vary in different parts of the world. In the UK, until recent years, most cases of scalp ringworm were the result of *M. canis* infection, usually acquired from cats, but immigration has led to the appearance of other scalp ringworm

organisms. In the USA, the usual causative organism is *T. tonsurans*, and in the Indian subcontinent the most common cause is *T. violaceum*.

One or more patches of partial hair loss develop on an otherwise normal scalp (Fig. 4.7). The affected scalp is scaly, and the hair is usually broken off just above the surface, producing irregular stubble. In some cases, there is little obvious inflammation, but in others this is prominent and there is pustule formation.

Occasionally the area of scalp involved is more extensive, producing an appearance suggestive of seborrhoeic dermatitis. *Microsporum canis* fluoresces yellow-green under long wavelength UV light (Wood's light)—see Chapter 2.

Kerion

Kerion (Greek, meaning 'honeycomb') is a term applied to severe inflammatory scalp ringworm, usually provoked by the fungus of cattle ringworm, but occasionally by other fungi. It resembles a bacterial infection, with pustules and abscesses (Fig. 4.8), and affected children are often given repeated courses of antibiotics on this assumption. They may also be subjected to surgical incision of the areas.

Cattle ringworm

In rural areas, young farm workers often suffer from cattle ringworm—older farmers have usually

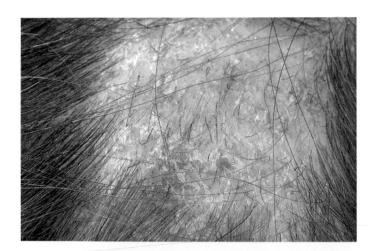

Figure 4.7 Scalp ringworm.

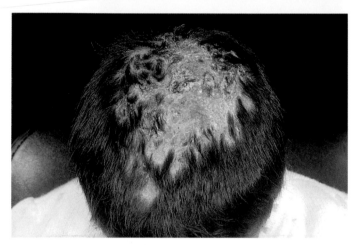

Figure 4.8 Kerion.

had the disease, and develop immunity against reinfection. The face and forearms are the areas most frequently affected. There is a marked inflammatory reaction to the fungus, producing an appearance resembling a bacterial infection (Fig. 4.9).

Children who visit farms may pick up the fungus from gates and fences where cattle have left keratin debris containing the organism, and subsequently develop a kerion.

Tinea incognito

This term is applied to a fungal infection whose appearance has been altered by inappropriate treatment with topical steroid preparations. Topical steroids suppress the inflammatory response to the fungus, and the typical scaly erythematous margin usually disappears, leaving an ill-defined area of patchy scaling erythema studded with pustules.

'Ide' reactions

Patients suffering from the florid vesicular type of athlete's foot may develop an acute vesiculobullous eruption on the hands known as an 'ide' reaction. The appearance is indistinguishable from the acute eczematous response known as pompholyx (see Chapter 7). The lesions on the hands do not contain fungus. The reaction appears to have an immunological basis, but the exact pathomechanism is unknown. Occasionally, a more

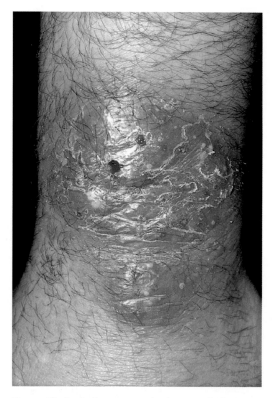

Figure 4.9 Cattle ringworm on the forearm of a farmer.

generalized maculopapular ide reaction accompanies a fungal infection.

Diagnosis

Skin scrapings, nail clippings and plucked hair can be examined, as described in Chapter 2. A little experience is necessary to distinguish fungal mycelium (Fig. 4.10) from cell walls and intercellular lipid, or filamentous debris. Fungal mycelium has the appearance of long rows of railway wagons which branch periodically. Material may also be sent to the mycology laboratory for culture.

Treatment

There are a number of topical antifungal agents available for the treatment of dermatophyte infections, including miconazole, clotrimazole, econazole, sulconazole and terbinafine. These can be used when small areas of skin are affected, but if a fungal infection is extensive it is preferable to employ an oral agent such as griseofulvin, terbinafine or itraconazole. Topical agents are not effective in scalp ringworm, and this should be treated with griseofulvin. Although terbinafine and itraconazole are also effective in scalp ringworm, they are at present not licensed for use in children in the UK. For skin and hair infections, griseofulvin should be given for a period of 4–6 weeks. In children, the dosage is calculated according to the child's weight (10 mg/kg); in adults the usual daily dose is 500 mg.

Skin infections may also be treated with terbinafine 250 mg daily for 2–4 weeks or itraconazole 100 mg daily for 15–30 days.

The treatment of choice for nail infections is oral terbinafine—250 mg daily for 6 weeks in fingernail infections and for 3 months in toenail infections. An alternative is itraconazole pulse therapy—200 mg twice daily for 7 days; for fingernails, repeat once after a 3-week drug-free interval; for toenails, repeat twice with a 3-week drug-free interval between each course. Various combination therapies, for example oral terbinafine plus topical amorolfine nail lacquer, have been suggested in attempts to increase cure rates and reduce costs of treatment.

Mycetoma (Madura foot)

In certain parts of the world, for example the Indian subcontinent, trauma to the feet may result in the inoculation of certain soil fungi, which produce a deep-seated chronic infection with abscesses and draining sinuses. The causative organisms are often unresponsive to systemic antifungal agents.

Candida infection

Candidiasis (moniliasis; 'thrush') is a term applied to infections of the skin and mucous membranes by yeast-like fungi of the genus *Candida*. The most common, *Candida albicans*, is a normal commensal of the human digestive tract, where it exists in balance with the bacterial flora. In its commensal role, *Candida* is present as budding yeasts. In a patho-

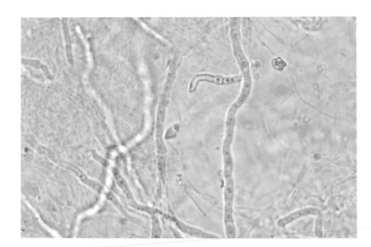

Figure 4.10 Fungal mycelium.

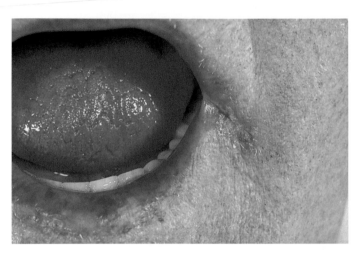

Figure 4.11 Angular cheilitis.

genic role, budding and mycelial forms are usually present. It only becomes pathogenic when situations favourable to its multiplication arise. These include topical and systemic steroid therapy, immune suppression of any aetiology (e.g. lymphoma, AIDS), broad-spectrum antibiotic therapy, diabetes mellitus, and the apposition of areas of skin to produce a warm, moist environment.

The diagnosis of candidiasis can be confirmed by culture of swabs taken from the affected areas.

Buccal mucosal candidiasis

White, curd-like plaques adhere to the buccal mucosa. If these are scraped off, the underlying epithelium is inflamed and friable. It may be treated with nystatin pastilles or oral suspension, amphotericin lozenges, miconazole oral gel or itraconazole liquid.

Angular cheilitis (perlèche)

Angular cheilitis is an inflammatory process occurring at the corners of the mouth (Fig. 4.11). The main factors involved in its causation, either alone or in combination, include infection with *Candida* or staphylococci, and the development of prominent creases at the angles of the mouth, either as a normal consequence of age, or in edentulous individuals who do not wear dentures or who have ill-fitting dentures. Saliva is drawn into the creases by capillary action, and salivary enzymes macerate the skin, producing sore, moist areas.

In denture wearers, modification of the dentures may help. Treatment with an imidazole/hydrocortisone combination, for example miconazole/hydrocortisone, is usually of benefit.

Chronic paronychia

This is a chronic inflammatory process affecting the proximal nail fold and nail matrix. It occurs predominantly in those whose hands are repeatedly immersed in water—housewives, bar staff, florists, fishmongers. A more widespread use of mechanical dishwashers, rather than the human variety, may be associated with a decline in the incidence of this disorder.

The clinical appearance is of thickening and erythema of the proximal nail fold ('bolstering'), and loss of the cuticle (Fig. 4.12). There is often an associated nail dystrophy. *Candida albicans* plays a pathogenic role, but bacteria may also be involved.

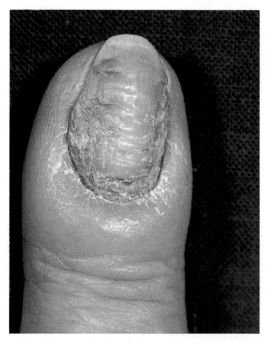

Figure 4.12 Chronic paronychia.

The absence of the cuticle allows access of irritant substances, such as detergents, to the area beneath the proximal nail fold, and this probably contributes to the inflammatory process.

This condition is quite distinct from acute bacterial paronychia, in which there is a short history, severe discomfort and ample production of green pus. Pressure on the swollen nail fold in chronic paronychia may produce a tiny bead of creamy pus from under the nail fold, but that is all.

Treatment consists of advice to keep the hands as dry as possible by wearing cotton-lined rubber or PVC gloves when working, and topical anti-*Candida* therapy, for example with an imidazole.

Balanitis/vulvovaginitis

Small white patches or eroded areas are present on the foreskin and glans of the uncircumcised penis. Predisposing factors are poor penile hygiene and diabetes mellitus. *Candida* balanitis may be a recurrent problem if a sexual partner has *Candida* vaginitis.

Candida vulvovaginitis presents with a creamy vaginal discharge and itchy erythema of the vulva. Pregnancy, oral contraceptives and diabetes mellitus are predisposing factors. Balanitis and vulvitis should be treated with a topical anti-*Candida* preparation, and there are several products available to treat vaginal candidiasis.

Don't forget to test the urine for sugar in anyone with *Candida* balanitis or vulvovaginitis.

Intertrigo

This is a term applied to maceration that occurs where two skin surfaces are in apposition—groins, axillae, submammary regions, or beneath an abdominal fat apron. Obesity and poor hygiene are contributory factors. *Candida* superinfection is often present, and is suggested clinically by the presence of creamy 'satellite' pustules at the margins of the affected areas. The pustules are easily ruptured, leaving a collarette of scale, and this gives a characteristic scalloped edge to the area of intertrigo.

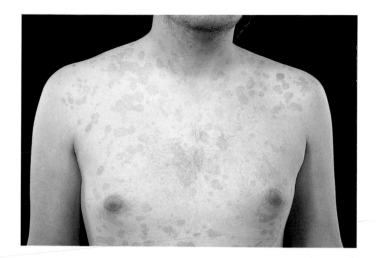

Figure 4.13 Pityriasis versicolor.

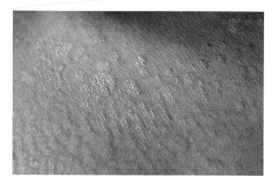

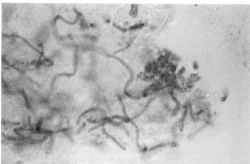

Figure 4.14 Close view of pityriasis versicolor showing fine 'branny' scale.

Figure 4.15 Spores and hyphae of *Malassezia* in pityriasis versicolor.

Therapy with a combined topical preparation containing an anti-*Candida* agent, such as miconazole, and hydrocortisone is usually beneficial, but attention to hygiene is also important.

Pityriasis versicolor

This condition occurs predominantly in young adults, and is caused by *Malassezia* yeasts, which are normal skin commensals present in pilosebaceous follicles. It is a common disorder in temperate zones and is seen even more frequently in tropical climates. The reason why these yeasts multiply and produce skin lesions in certain individuals is unknown.

On a fair skin, the lesions are light-brown macules with a fine surface scale (Figs 4.13 & 4.14), and

they occur predominantly on the trunk and upper arms. They are usually asymptomatic, but are a cosmetic nuisance. On pigmented skin, the typical appearance is of patchy hypopigmentation. The loss of pigment is thought to be related to production of azelaic acid by the yeasts that inhibits tyrosinase and thereby interferes with melanin production. The colour variation, depending on the background skin colour, is the reason for the 'versicolor' in the name.

The diagnosis can be confirmed by microscopic examination of skin scrapings in a mixture of 10% potassium hydroxide and Parker Quink ink (Fig. 4.15), when characteristic clumps of round spores and short, stubby hyphae can be seen (an appearance which has been called 'spaghetti and meatballs').

A simple treatment is selenium sulfide, in the form of a shampoo (Selsun), left on the skin for a few minutes during bathing. This will usually clear the organism in 2–3 weeks. Topical imidazole antifungal creams and ketoconazole shampoo are also effective against *Malassezia*, as is topical terbinafine. Oral itraconazole is an alternative (200 mg daily for 7 days). Griseofulvin and oral terbinafine are ineffective.

Pityriasis versicolor tends to recur, and treatment may have to be repeated. Hypopigmented areas may take a considerable time to repigment, and their persistence should not be taken as evidence of treatment failure.

Chapter 5

Ectoparasite infections

Scabies

There's a squeak of pure delight from a matey little mite,

As it tortuously tunnels in the skin,

Singing furrow, folly furrow, come and join me in my burrow,

And we'll view the epidermis from within

    (Guy's *Acarus*)

Aetiology

Scabies (Latin = the scab, mange, itch) is caused by small, eight-legged mites (*Sarcoptes scabiei*), and is acquired by close physical contact with another individual suffering from the disease—prolonged hand holding is probably the usual means of spread. Any age group may be affected. It is common in children and young adults, and in recent years has become frequent in elderly people, usually in a residential care home environment. Transient contact is not sufficient for spread, and anyone encountering ordinary cases of scabies in a healthcare setting should not be afraid of acquiring the disease.

The female scabies mite burrows in the epidermis, and lays eggs in the burrow behind her. Male scabies mites have but one function in life, and after the chase and the consummation they expire. Initially, the host is unaware of the mining activity in the epidermis, but after a period of 4–6 weeks hypersensitivity to the mite or its products develops, and itching begins. The asymptomatic period is obviously very useful to the parasite because it has time to establish itself before the host response develops. Thereafter, life becomes hazardous for the mites because burrows will be excoriated and mites and eggs destroyed. In this way, the host keeps the mite population in check, and in most individuals suffering from scabies the average number of adult female mites on the skin is no more than a dozen.

Clinical features

The patient complains of itching, which is characteristically worse at night. Scabies should be considered in anyone presenting with this history.

There are two principal types of skin lesion in scabies—burrows and the scabies 'rash'. Burrows are found principally on the hands and feet—the sides of the fingers and toes, the toe-web spaces, the wrists and the insteps. In infants, burrows are often present on the palms of the hands and soles of the feet, and may also be present on the trunk and the head and neck. Burrows on the trunk are a common finding in elderly patients and they may also occur on the head and neck. Each burrow is several millimetres long, usually tortuous, with a vesicle at one end adjacent to the burrowing mite, and often surrounded by mild erythema (Fig. 5.1). Burrows also occur on the male genitalia, usually

41

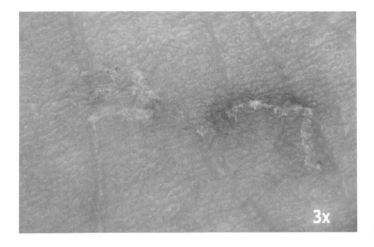

Figure 5.1 Typical scabies burrow.

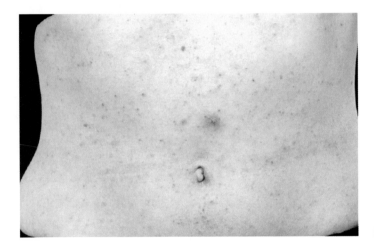

Figure 5.2 The scabies 'rash'.

surmounting inflammatory papules, and these papules on the penis and scrotum are pathognomonic of scabies. If scabies is suspected in a male, the genitalia should always be examined.

The 'rash' of scabies is an eruption of tiny inflammatory papules that occur mainly around the axillae and umbilicus, and on the thighs (Fig. 5.2). The rash is an allergic reaction to the mites.

In addition to these primary skin lesions, there may be secondary changes such as excoriations, eczematization and secondary bacterial infection. In some parts of the world, secondary infection of scabies lesions with nephritogenic streptococci is associated with the development of poststreptococcal glomerulonephritis.

Diagnosis

Absolute confirmation of the diagnosis can only be made by demonstrating the mites or eggs microscopically. In order to do this, burrows must be found, and this usually requires some expertise. Look carefully, in good light, at the hands and feet. A magnifying glass may be of some help, but myopia is a distinct advantage. Once a burrow, or a suspected burrow, has been identified, it should be gently scraped off the skin with the edge of a scalpel blade—dermatologists sometimes use a blunt scalpel known as a 'banana' scalpel for this task. The scrapings should be placed on a microscope slide with a few drops of 10% KOH, covered

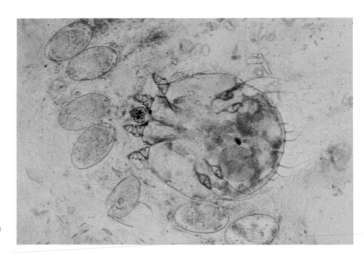

Figure 5.3 Scabies mite and eggs in potassium hydroxide preparation.

with a coverslip and examined under the microscope. The presence of mites, eggs or even egg shells confirms the diagnosis (Fig. 5.3). Do not attempt to scrape any lesions on the penis—the proximity of a scalpel to this area leads to understandable apprehension, and is in any case rarely rewarded by the demonstration of mites.

A dermatoscope is a useful tool for viewing mites *in situ* in their burrows.

Treatment

Scabies is treated by eating young alligators and washing the skin with urine. (Mexican Folk Medicine)

It is important to explain to patients precisely how to use their treatment, and written explanatory treatment sheets are useful. All family members, and close physical contacts of an affected individual, should be treated simultaneously. Topical agents should be applied from the neck to the toes, and patients should be reminded not to wash their hands after applying treatment. In infants, elderly and immunocompromised patients, in whom burrows can occur on the head and neck, it may be necessary to extend application to these areas. Itching does not resolve immediately following treatment, but will improve gradually over 2–3 weeks as the superficial epidermis, containing the allergenic mites, is shed. A topical antipruritic such

as crotamiton 10% with hydrocortisone 0.25% can be used on residual itchy areas. It is not necessary to 'disinfest' clothing and soft furnishings—laundering of underwear and nightclothes is all that is required.

Available treatments

Malathion 0.5%
Aqueous preparations are preferred because they do not irritate excoriated or eczematized skin. Wash off after 24 h.

5% Permethrin cream
Wash off after 8–12 h.

A single application of malathion or permethrin is often effective, but a second application 7 days later is recommended.

Benzyl benzoate emulsion
Although superseded by malathion and permethrin in some parts of the world, in many countries benzyl benzoate is still used to treat scabies because it is effective and inexpensive. One regimen involves three applications in a 24-h period. On the evening of day 1 apply the emulsion from the neck to the toes. Allow to dry, then apply a second coat. The following morning apply a third coat, and then wash off the benzyl benzoate on the evening of day 2. Treatment is then complete, and this

should be stressed to the patient because repeated use will produce an irritant dermatitis.

Irritancy is its main drawback.

Treatment of infants

As burrows can occur on the head and neck, it may be necessary to extend application of topical therapy to these areas. The treatment of choice is permethrin.

Because of the availability of non-irritant agents, benzyl benzoate is not recommended for use in infants, but if it is employed it should be diluted to reduce its irritancy.

Treatment in pregnancy

There is understandable concern about potential toxic effects on the fetus of scabicides when used in pregnancy. However, there is no definitive evidence that any of the currently employed topical scabicides has been responsible for harmful effects in pregnancy following appropriate use. Hence, in the absence of evidence of fetal toxicity, use of malathion or permethrin appears to be safe.

Crusted (Norwegian) scabies

This is an uncommon type of scabies in which enormous numbers of mites are present in crusted lesions on the skin. It was called Norwegian scabies because it was originally described in Norwegian lepers, but the term 'crusted' is now preferred. The mite is exactly the same as that causing ordinary scabies. Mites are present in such huge numbers because of an altered host response to their presence. Crusted scabies may develop when itching is not perceived because of sensory loss from neurological disorders (hence its occurrence in lepers), in individuals who are immunosuppressed, either as a result of disease (e.g. AIDS) or treatment (e.g. systemic steroids; organ transplantation), or when patients are unable to scratch because of severe rheumatoid arthritis or paresis. In these circumstances, when the host does not itch or cannot scratch, burrows are not destroyed and the mite population multiplies unchecked. Crusted scabies also occurs more frequently in individuals with Down's syndrome.

The crusted skin lesions can contain millions of mites and eggs, and these are shed into the environment on flakes of keratin. Anyone coming into contact with a patient suffering from crusted scabies is at risk of acquiring ordinary scabies, and undiagnosed cases may be responsible for outbreaks of scabies in hospitals and residential homes.

Clinical features

The hands and feet are usually encased in a thick, fissured crust, and areas of crusting may be present on other parts of the body, including the head and neck. The nails are often grossly thickened (Fig. 5.4). The changes may resemble psoriatic scaling or

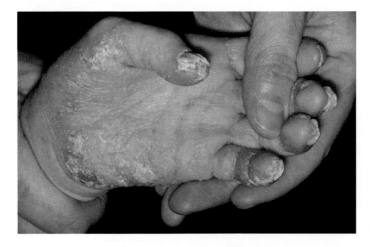

Figure 5.4 Crusted scabies in a youth with Down's syndrome.

hyperkeratotic eczema, and this can lead to the diagnosis being missed. Burrows are usually impossible to identify in the crusted areas, but may be found on less severely affected parts of the body. Microscopy of the scales reveals numerous mites and eggs.

Treatment

The patient should be isolated, and nurses responsible for the patient's care should wear gowns and gloves. All medical staff and carers, and any other individuals who have been in contact with the patient before diagnosis and treatment, should be treated with a topical scabicide.

Crusted scabies is often difficult to cure with topical agents, and usually requires several applications of a scabicide. Treatment should be applied to the whole body, including the head and neck. Oral ivermectin given as a single dose of 200 µg per kg body weight is an effective treatment, and higher cure rates have been obtained by giving two doses separated by an interval of 7 days, particularly in immunosuppressed individuals. It is usually combined with a topical scabicide. Ivermectin is not licensed for use in the treatment of scabies in humans, but may be obtained on a named-patient basis from the manufacturer. It has been used for many years as a treatment for onchocerciasis (river blindness) and other types of filariasis, and is employed in veterinary practice to deal with several types of animal parasites.

Institutional outbreaks of scabies

The huge increase in the number of residential care and nursing homes for elderly people in the UK in recent years has been associated with numerous outbreaks of scabies in these facilities. Although some are related to cases of crusted scabies, others appear to originate from residents who have a large mite population, or from infected carers. Close contact between residents and carers in these homes is common—carers usually hold the hands of residents to provide support when walking, and this facilitates spread of the disease.

All residents, their carers and the carers' families should be treated with a topical scabicide. Residents who have very numerous burrows, or are suffering from crusted scabies, will require more intensive treatment and preferably should be isolated until cured. If such individuals are not identified, there is a risk that they may only partially respond to treatment and therefore provide a source for a further outbreak. Ivermectin may prove to be of value in dealing with outbreaks of scabies in residential homes and similar communities.

Pediculosis

Head lice (*Pediculus capitis*)

Her ladyship said when I went to her house,
That she did not esteem me three skips of a louse;
I freely forgave what the dear creature said,
For ladies will talk of what runs in their head.
(Theodore Hook)

Head lice are wingless insects that live on the scalp, and feed on blood. Adult head lice are 2–4 mm in length. They are acquired by head-to-head contact with another infected individual. It is still a commonly held belief that head lice are associated with poor hygiene, perhaps supported by the findings of surveys in the earlier part of the twentieth century which showed that head louse infection was principally a problem of the lower classes in large industrial conurbations. However, in more recent years, the head louse has climbed the social ladder and taken up rural pursuits, and is now widely distributed in all socioeconomic groups.

The adult female louse lays eggs which she cements to hair shafts (Fig. 5.5). The eggs are flesh coloured and are difficult to see, but once the louse nymph has emerged (after about 10 days) the empty egg case (nit) is more readily visible.

Clinical features

Itching is the main symptom. Nits tend to be more numerous in the occipital region of the scalp and above the ears (Fig. 5.6). Occasionally, flakes of

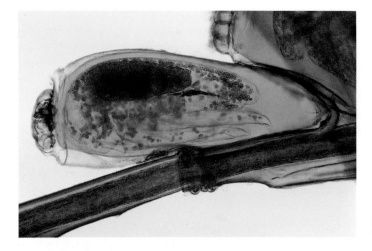

Figure 5.5 Head louse eggs cemented to a hair shaft.

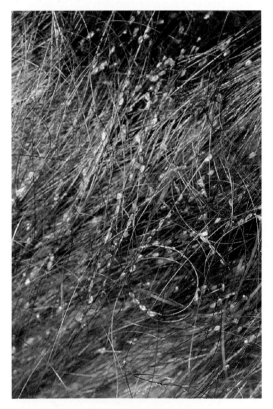

Figure 5.6 Head louse eggs and egg cases.

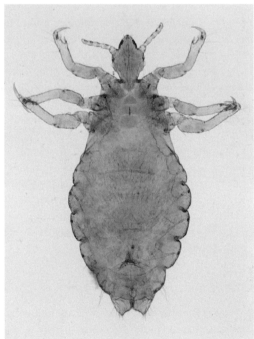

Figure 5.7 The head louse.

dandruff or keratin casts around hair shafts may be mistaken for nits, but the distinction is obvious if the material is examined microscopically. Adult lice and nymphs will be found without difficulty in heavier infections (Fig. 5.7). Impetigo may occur as a result of inoculation of staphylococci into the skin during scratching; the term 'nitwit' is derived from the substandard performance of children who had large head louse populations, secondary skin sepsis and probably also anaemia, and were chronically unwell as a result.

Treatment

The approach to treatment has changed in recent years, and it is now considered appropriate to employ a strategy that includes both physical and chemical methods. Chemical means of control, employing insecticides, have been widely used throughout the world. Insecticides are easy to use and convenient, and they have proved very effective. However, there is concern about potential adverse effects, particularly from residual insecticides such as lindane (which is no longer used in some parts of the world, including the UK), not only on humans but also on the environment. In addition, there is evidence of widespread resistance of head lice to malathion and pyrethroid insecticides.

Pediculicides

- Malathion
- Carbaryl
- Synthetic pyrethroids:
  permethrin
  phenothrin

Preparations with an aqueous basis are less likely than those with an alcohol basis to irritate an excoriated scalp, they do not irritate the bronchi of asthmatics, and they are not flammable. None of these insecticides is fully ovicidal, and treatment should therefore be repeated after 7–10 days in order to kill any louse nymphs emerging from surviving eggs.

Several over-the-counter head louse treatments contain tea-tree or lavender oil, and there is anecdotal evidence that they are effective. However, they have not been formally assessed in clinical trials.

A simple physical method of treatment involves washing the hair with an ordinary shampoo followed by the application of generous quantities of conditioner. The hair is then combed with a fine-toothed comb with closely set teeth, which removes any lice. This process is repeated every 4 days for 2 weeks.

Clothing lice (*Pediculus humanus*)

The louse
Has very little 'nous',
Its only pursuit
Is the hirsute.
(I. Kenvyn Evans)

The clothing or body louse is a parasite that thrives in association with poverty and poor hygiene. It lives on, and lays its eggs in the seams of, clothing, and only moves onto the body to feed on blood. It is still common in the poorer countries of the world, but in an affluent society its usual hosts are down-and-outs and vagrants who have only one set of clothes that are never removed or cleaned. An individual who regularly changes clothing and maintains a reasonable standard of hygiene will never harbour clothing lice because the lice will not survive laundering and ironing of garments. Clothing lice are vectors of epidemic typhus, a rickettsial disease that has been responsible for millions of deaths over the centuries.

Clinical features

Clothing lice usually provoke itching, and their host is often covered in excoriations. The itching appears to be the result of an acquired hypersensitivity to louse salivary antigens. If clothing louse infection is suspected, there is no point in searching the patient for lice—you may be lucky and find an occasional louse at lunch on the body, but it is the clothing you should examine (Fig. 5.8).

Treatment

All the patient requires is a bath. A complete change of clean clothing should be supplied and the infested clothing either destroyed or laundered at temperatures of 60°C or above. Dry cleaning or use of a tumble drier are alternatives.

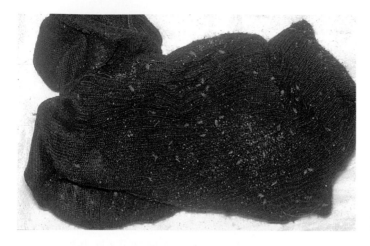

Figure 5.8 Clothing lice and eggs residing in a sock.

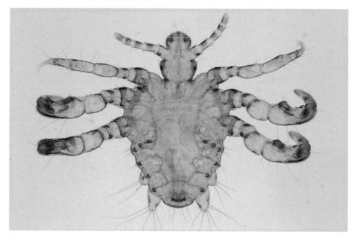

Figure 5.9 The crab louse.

Crab lice (*Pthirus pubis*)

It's no good standing on the seat
The crabs in here can jump 10 feet.
If you think that's rather high,
Go next door, the buggers fly!
(Toilet graffito)

Crab lice, also known as pubic lice and love bugs, and in France as *papillons d'amour*, are usually transmitted during close physical contact with an infected individual, in spite of the above allegation of contagion from toilet seats. At one time they were thought to be rather sedentary lice, but experiments subsequently demonstrated that when its host is sleeping the crab louse becomes quite ac-

tive. It is a louse adapted to living in hair of a particular density. It cannot colonize scalp hair, except at the margins of the scalp, but pubic, axillary, beard and eyelash hair are perfectly acceptable to it, and in an extremely hairy male most of the body may resemble a crab louse adventure playground. The crab louse is so named because of its squat shape and powerful claws, resembling a crab's pincers (Fig. 5.9), with which it grasps hair. Female crab lice, like head lice, stick their eggs to hair shafts with a cement material.

Clinical features

Itching, usually nocturnal, is the symptom that draws the host's attention to these little passen-

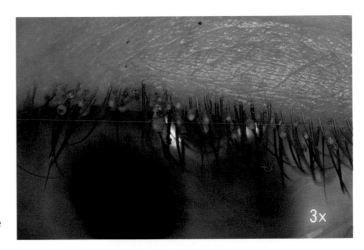

3x

Figure 5.10 Crab louse eggs on the eyelashes.

gers. Self-examination then reveals the reason for the itch, and the doctor is often presented with a folded piece of paper containing 'specimens'. When folded paper is opened, it has a tendency to flick its contents in all directions, leaving the unlucky recipient anxiously awaiting signs of personal contamination for weeks thereafter.

Lice are usually visible on the affected areas, but sometimes their eggs, which are a brown colour, are easier to see. If the parasites are very numerous, the underclothes may be speckled with spots of altered blood excreted by the lice. Lice on the eyelids festoon the lashes with their eggs (Fig. 5.10). Children may acquire crab lice as a result of normal close physical contact with an infected parent. The lice will colonize the eyelashes and scalp margin. As an isolated finding, crab louse infection in a child should not be considered indicative of sexual abuse.

Treatment

The same pediculicides that are used to eradicate head lice are effective against crab lice, but aqueous preparations should be used because alcohol-based preparations will irritate the scrotum. The whole body should be treated, including the scalp if there is evidence of lice on the scalp margins. Sexual contacts should also be treated. The treatment should be repeated after an interval of 7–10 days.

Eyelash infection may be treated by the application of white soft paraffin (Vaseline) three times a day for 2–3 weeks. This acts by blocking the louse respiratory system, thereby suffocating the insects.

Papular urticaria

Often referred to as 'heat bumps' by patients, papular urticaria is a typical response to the bites of a number of arthropods, including biting flies, mosquitoes, mites, fleas and bed bugs. The lesions are small urticated papules (Fig. 5.11), usually grouped (sometimes in groups of three, fancifully labelled 'breakfast, lunch and dinner'), and they may be surmounted by a tiny vesicle. They are so itchy that their tops are rapidly excoriated. They develop as a result of a hypersensitivity response to antigens in the arthropods' saliva. Eventually, in many people, immunological tolerance to the antigens develops and they subsequently do not react to the bites.

Fleas

May the fleas of a thousand camels infest your armpits! (Arab curse)

The most common cause of papular urticaria acquired in the home environment is flea bites. It is not the human flea, *Pulex irritans*, which is responsible, but fleas whose natural hosts are household pets. A familiar clinical picture is of multiple

49

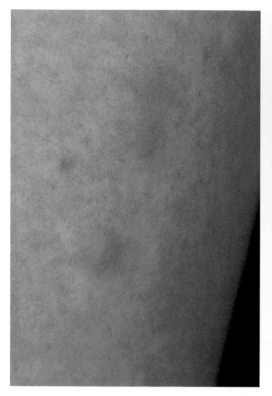

Figure 5.11 Papular urticaria.

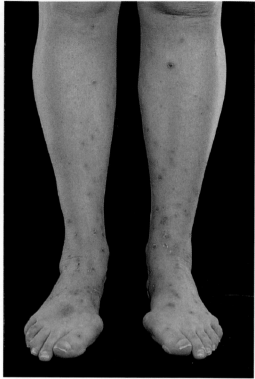

Figure 5.12 Flea bites on the ankles.

lesions, some of which may form blisters, around the ankles of women (Fig. 5.12). Men are rarely affected, because socks and trousers deny fleas access to the ankles.

Cats and dogs are perambulating quadripedal 'meals-on-wheels' for the fleas (Fig. 5.13). However, although fleas are present on the animals, their numbers are small in comparison with the fleas in various stages of development scattered throughout the household. Flea eggs are not sticky, and when laid by fleas feeding on an animal they drop out of the coat into the surroundings—the cat-basket, the carpet, the sofa or the counterpane. Eggs, larvae, pupae and adult fleas are present in all these areas. Hence, the house should be treated, as well as the pets. There are commercially available preparations designed to be sprayed around the house on carpets and soft furnishings, and veterinary products to be applied topically or fed to the animal, usually containing synthetic equivalents

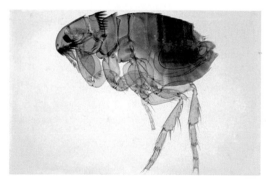

Figure 5.13 A cat flea.

of insect growth regulatory hormones that interfere with flea development.

Occasionally, bird fleas will gain access to homes from nests under the eaves, and may be responsible for more extensive lesions of papular urticaria.

Bed bugs (*Cimex lectularius*)

The butterfly has wings of gold,
The firefly wings of flame,
The bed bug has no wings at all,
But he gets there just the same.

Perhaps this rhyme relates to the, probably inaccurate, tale that if one attempts to stop bed bugs crawling up bed legs at night by placing the legs in bowls of water, the cunning bugs climb the walls, cross the ceiling and drop on the occupants of the bed from above.

Bed bugs are not the most appealing of creatures. They live in dilapidated housing behind peeling wallpaper and rotten skirting boards, and emerge an hour or so before dawn to feed on the sleeping occupants of bedrooms. They feed on blood and, although the process of feeding does not cause the host any pain, a reaction to the bites of the bugs usually results in papular urticaria or bullous lesions. These insects are 5–6mm long, dark brown in colour, and can move quite rapidly. Fortunately, bed-bug infestation of houses in developed countries is now uncommon, but if it is suspected the local environmental health department should be asked to inspect and disinfest the property.

Animal mites

Human contact with animals suffering from sarcoptic mange may result in the development of scattered itchy papules, often on areas coming into contact with the animals—for example, the abdomen and thighs if a mangy dog sits on its owner's lap. It is highly unlikely that these animal mites will establish themselves on humans, because they are species specific, but there have been a few reports in which it is said to have occurred.

Dogs, cats and rabbits are the natural hosts of *Cheyletiella* mites, and these may cause skin lesions in humans. Dogs are the usual culprits. On the animal, the mites provoke a heavy scurf over the back (known in veterinary circles as 'walking dandruff'), but hardly bother it otherwise. On the owner, itchy papules appear principally on the abdomen, but occasionally also on the thighs and arms—sites of contact with the animal. The diagnosis can be confirmed by taking combings from the animal's coat and demonstrating the mite microscopically. Once the animal has been treated by a veterinary practitioner the human skin lesions resolve spontaneously.

Bird mites may gain access to houses from nests under the eaves, and can cause itchy papular lesions.

Ticks

Ixodid, or hard ticks, are very common, particularly in wooded areas where there are deer populations. They feed on blood, and their barbed mouthparts are held in the skin of the host during feeding by a protein cement material. If a tick is pulled off the skin abruptly, its mouthparts may be left *in situ*, and will provoke a foreign-body reaction.

Ixodid ticks are vectors of Lyme disease which is caused by the spirochaete *Borrelia burgdorferi*. Lyme disease (named after the town in Connecticut where its association with ticks was first discovered) affects the skin, joints, central nervous system and the heart. It responds to treatment with benzylpenicillin, amoxicillin (amoxycillin) or tetracyclines.

Probably the best way to remove a tick is to grasp it as close to the skin as possible with fine tweezers or forceps, and exert gentle continuous traction.

Chapter 6

Acne, acneiform eruptions and rosacea

Out, damned spot! Out, I say! (Shakespeare, *Macbeth* v.i)

Introduction

This chapter deals with disorders which cause papules and pustules, often known in the vernacular as 'spots' or 'zits'. Some are aetiologically related and can properly be called variants of acne (a corruption of the Greek *akme*—a point). Others produce lesions closely or superficially resembling 'true' acne: the acneiform disorders and rosacea. A summary of the 'acne family' is given below.

The acne family
Acne vulgaris
• 'Classical'
• Infantile and juvenile onset
• Late onset
• Severe (acne conglobata; nodulocystic)
• With systemic symptoms (acne fulminans)
Secondary acne
• Endocrine associated
• Medicaments
• Oils
• Chloracne
Hidradenitis suppurativa

Acne vulgaris and its variants

Acne vulgaris

About 80% of people develop some spottiness. Acne may be very mild indeed, but at its most severe, gross and unsightly changes are seen.

Acne may be associated with underlying endocrinological abnormalities (see below) but usually it is not.

Age of onset and course

The first problems are usually encountered in adolescence, although there are exceptions (see below).

Lesions of acne vary considerably with time. Most patients notice marked fluctuations in the number and severity of spots, and in girls this is often related to the menstrual cycle. The condition frequently deteriorates at times of stress.

Acne usually gets worse for a while before gradually settling after 2–3 years, and usually disappearing altogether. The peak of severity is earlier in girls than in boys. In some individuals, the time-course may be much more prolonged, with lesions continuing to develop well into adult life.

There are two groups, described below, in whom true acne develops outside adolescence.

Infantile/juvenile acne

Typical acne is occasionally seen in infants and children (especially boys), usually at 3–12 months of age. Although lesions subside after 4–5 years, adolescence often heralds a severe recrudescence. Endocrine abnormalities are very rare, but should be considered, especially in a girl with signs of virilism.

Late-onset acne

A number of women and some men develop acne in their twenties and beyond. In women, this is often with marked premenstrual exacerbations. Endocrinological investigation is generally unrewarding, but polycystic ovary syndrome is an important exception.

The psychological impact of acne

Acne can make life miserable, and its predilection for the teens and twenties means that its effects are on those least well equipped to cope.

The face is prominently involved, and in adolescence the face assumes increasing importance as self-image develops. At the time when acne strikes, major relationships outside the family and close circles of same-sex friends are increasingly crucial. Realize, too, that the psychological impact of acne is not necessarily related to the degree of severity as perceived by an outsider. A young person may spend just as long staring miserably into the mirror when there are only a few spots as when there are hundreds.

Clinical features

Physical signs

The characteristic distribution is as follows.

> **Site and distribution of acne**
>
> - Face, any part of which may be involved
> - Neck, especially posteriorly
> - Ears
> - Upper back
> - Anterior chest, in an inverted 'V' from the shoulders to the xiphisternum
> - Shoulders

In severe acne, lesions may extend down the arms, across the whole of the central back, and onto the buttocks.

The appearance of the skin

The first physical sign to note is that the face and upper trunk become very greasy (Fig. 6.1) due to increased production of sebum. This is normal at puberty, but is excessive in those with acne. Scalp hair is often very greasy too. Greasiness alone may be bad enough for the patient to seek advice.

The individual lesions of acne

A cardinal feature is that there are several different types of lesion at any one time.

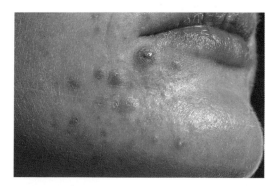

Figure 6.1 This girl's face shows the typical greasy skin of the acne sufferer, in addition to papules and pustules.

Acne vulgaris lesions

- Comedones:
  closed ('whiteheads')
  open ('blackheads')
- Papules
- Pustules
- Nodules
- Cysts
- Scars

Comedones (singular: comedo)

The presence of comedones is an important diagnostic aid. There are two types: closed (or 'whitehead') and open (or 'blackhead').

Closed comedones are more easily felt than seen. They are very small papules, with a central point or elevation (Fig. 6.2). They are often most numerous on the forehead and cheeks. There is little or no inflammation.

Open comedones (blackheads) are dilated, blocked hair follicles, but it is not clear what causes the characteristic black dots. Burnt-out inflammatory lesions may leave multiheaded blackheads, particularly on the shoulders and upper trunk. Blackheads are virtually pathognomonic of acne in the younger patient (although advanced solar damage may also result in blackhead formation).

Papules and pustules

The majority of patients with acne develop papules and pustules. They are the well-known little red spots or pustules on a red base. They may itch or be quite painful. Papules develop rapidly, often over a few hours, and frequently become pustular as they evolve. They resolve over the course of a few days. New lesions may arise in exactly the same site on many occasions.

Nodules and cysts

With increasing severity, and as the inflammation extends deeper, the size of visible and palpable lesions increases, resulting in deep-seated nodules and cysts (Figs 6.3 & 6.4). Many patients develop a few, but some have large numbers: a situation in which the term 'acne conglobata' is used.

Such lesions are often extremely uncomfortable and last much longer than more superficial changes. Some become chronic, and may result in permanent cyst formation (see Chapter 9).

Scars

The final common pathway for the inflammatory process of acne is scarring, which will remain as a lifetime's legacy of adolescent anguish. Character-

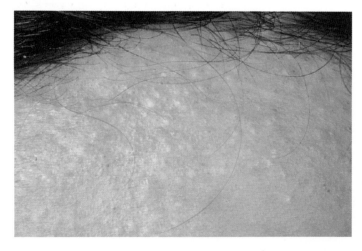

Figure 6.2 Closed comedones.

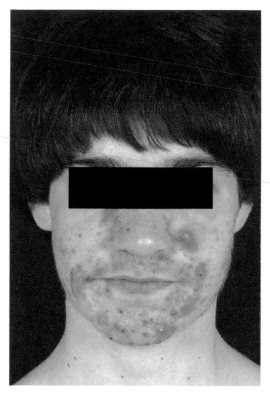

Figure 6.3 Acne conglobata.

istically, small, deep 'ice-pick' scars occur, but more severe disease can leave gross changes, with atrophy (Fig. 6.5) or keloid formation (see Chapter 9).

Systemic symptoms (acne fulminans)

Very occasionally a young man (almost always) develops severe nodulocystic acne accompanied by fever, malaise and joint pain and swelling. This is known as 'acne fulminans'.

Pathogenesis of acne

The aetio-pathology of acne remains to be elucidated fully. However, several key features may contribute to the final picture (see Fig. 6.6), although this does not fully explain every aspect of the disorder: the occurrence of prepubertal acne, for example.

Pathogenesis of acne

1 Androgens (usually in normal amounts) stimulate increased sebum production
2 Hair follicles with particularly large sebaceous glands (on the face, neck, chest and back) become blocked by hyperkeratosis
3 This results in the closed comedo
4 Within the follicle, an obligate anaerobe (*Propionibacterium acnes*) proliferates
5 This organism acts on sebum, releasing inflammatory chemicals
6 These leak into the surrounding dermis
7 The body mounts an intense acute inflammatory response. The result of this is the papule, pustule or nodule

As the inflammation subsides, a variable amount of fibrosis occurs. This may produce scarring, particularly if repeated episodes occur in the same site. Sometimes epithelial remnants become walled off by fibrosis, producing cysts.

Treatment of acne

Topical therapies

Many over-the-counter remedies rely on sulfur and other astringents which make the skin flaky and unblock hair follicles.

Topical antiseptics such as povidone iodine and chlorhexidine are often prescribed, but are of little proven value.

Benzoyl peroxide is widely used. It reduces comedones but must be used regularly and in the long term. There are several strengths: start with a weak preparation, applied once daily, and gradually progress to higher concentrations.

Vitamin A derivatives (retinoids) and retinoid-like agents also reduce comedones. Preparations in this category include retinoic acid, isotretinoin (13-*cis*-retinoic acid) and adapalene. All work well but can be irritant.

Topical tetracyclines, erythromycin and clindamycin are available, and are generally applied once daily. All have been shown to be useful in milder acne. There are some preparations that combine antibiotics with other agents such as benzoyl peroxide.

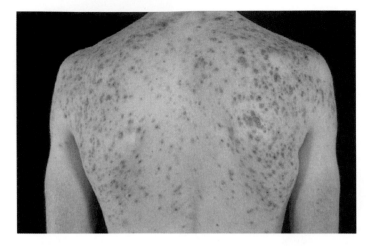

Figure 6.4 Severe acne on the back.

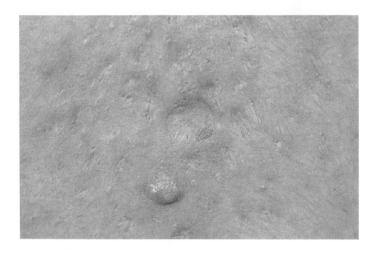

Figure 6.5 Atrophic scarring in acne.

Treatments for acne

Topical
- Benzoyl peroxide
- Retinoids and retinoid-like agents
- Sulfur and astringents
- Topical antiseptics, antibiotics and combination products

Systemic
- Antibiotics
- Cyproterone acetate
- 13-*cis*-retinoic acid (isotretinoin)
- Steroids

Surgical intervention

Systemic therapies

Antibiotics are the mainstay of the treatment of papulopustular acne. It is not known precisely how they work, but they reduce bacterial counts, at least initially, and may also have direct anti-inflammatory effects.

The most effective are the tetracyclines, erythromycin and trimethoprim. To work, antibiotics must be fat soluble, and the *penicillins are therefore useless*. Most tetracyclines should be taken on an empty stomach. Tetracyclines are contraindicated in children under 12, and in pregnant or lactating women.

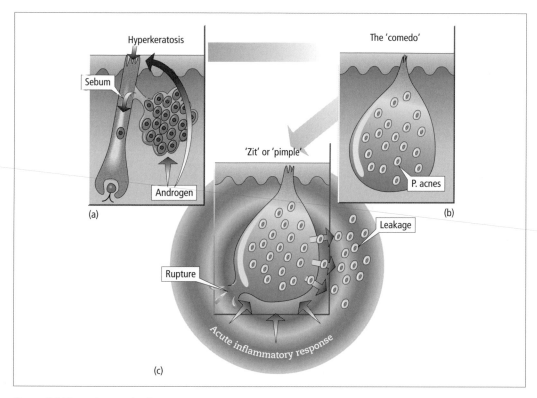

Figure 6.6 The pathogenesis of acne.

Cyproterone acetate is an antiandrogen which can only be given to women. It is given along with oestrogen to prevent menorrhagia and to ensure contraceptive cover (it will feminize a male fetus). Its effect is rather slow.

13-*cis*-retinoic acid (isotretinoin) is a highly effective oral vitamin A derivative which dramatically reduces sebum production. Isotretinoin is only available on hospital prescription in the UK. Over 90% of patients have complete clearance of their acne and in up to 80% there is no relapse. It has several side-effects: dry lips, eyes and skin, nosebleeds, mild alopecia, aches and pains. It also raises blood fat levels and may affect liver function tests. The most serious problem is teratogenicity. Female patients must not become pregnant when taking isotretinoin, as it will produce fetal abnormalities. All female patients must therefore be monitored very carefully throughout treatment. In the UK clinicians and patients should adhere to an agreed 'Pregnancy Prevention Protocol'. The drug has also developed a reputation for causing psychological disturbances. Whether this is a significant causal effect remains controversial, but all patients should be warned about mood changes, especially depression.

Dapsone may also be a useful addition in patients with very troublesome acne, and is safe.

Steroids can be used intralesionally or systemically in severe acne (they are virtually always needed in acne fulminans).

Surgical intervention

Simple measures, such as removing multiple comedones with a comedone extractor, may improve the appearance. It certainly gives great pleasure and satisfaction to a girl- or boyfriend who likes to pop out blackheads! Large, residual cysts may need to be excised, but there is a risk of keloid scarring.

Plastic surgeons can sometimes help acne scarring by dermabrasion, but this must not be attempted until the acne is fully under control.

Management of a patient with acne

The approach to treatment must be tailored to the individual, but there are some helpful guidelines. Let's first dispel some myths!

Common acne myths

- Acne is due to fatty food or sweets
- Acne is due to being dirty
- Acne is due to 'hormonal imbalance'
- Acne is related to sexual behaviour
All rubbish!
- Diet plays no role at all; there is no need to avoid sweets, chocolate or chips
- Even hourly washing would make no difference
- Hormones are normal in the vast majority
- Neither too little, nor too much sex makes any difference (thank goodness!)

Assessment of the patient

It can be useful to consider acne in three broad severity bands: mild, moderate and severe.

Mild acne may respond to topical treatment alone. Begin with benzoyl peroxide, retinoic acid, isotretinoin or adapalene, and/or a topical antibiotic. An antibiotic/benzoyl peroxide combination can be a useful option.

Moderate acne should initially be treated with a combination of a topical agent and oral oxytetracycline or erythromycin in a dose of 500 mg twice daily. Continue for at least 3–6 months before reassessing. Alternative tetracyclines have their advocates: some may be better absorbed or tolerated, but most are more expensive and there is generally no indication for their use as first-line agents.

If the response is not satisfactory, the acne should be managed as outlined below.

Severe acne may be controlled to some extent by systemic antibiotics, but this degree of acne often demands more aggressive treatment. Girls may respond to cyproterone acetate with or without antibiotics, allowing at least 6 months for a response.

Dapsone at a dose of 25 mg twice daily can be helpful.

However, any girls and most young men with severe or persistent acne eventually require isotretinoin, usually for 4–6 months. The daily dose may begin at 0.5 mg/kg but may need to be raised to 1 mg/kg.

Intralesional steroids are useful for acute inflammatory lesions. Very rarely, systemic steroid therapy may be required, especially in acne fulminans.

Surgical intervention may be required later to help overcome the devastation wreaked by this degree of acne.

Acne assessment

Mild
Only comedones *and/or* only a few papulopustular lesions restricted to the face

Moderate
More papulopustular lesions on the face or over a wider area *and/or* occasional nodules

Severe
Very widespread papulopustular lesions *and/or* nodulocystic lesions *and/or* systemic symptoms
or acne of moderate severity, failing to settle within 6 months of therapy
or acne of whatever severity with significant psychological upset

---

Secondary acne

Acne lesions may arise as a consequence of other primary pathological processes. Such 'secondary' acne is often monomorphic and generally mild.

An exception is acne occurring in patients with *endocrine abnormalities*. The most common is polycystic ovary syndrome, in which acne of any severity may accompany hirsutism, menstrual irregularities and infertility. Any cause of abnormally high circulating androgen levels (such as tumours) may also cause quite severe acne, while lesions in Cushing's syndrome are milder.

Medicaments such as greasy ointments, pomades and topical steroids may induce comedones and occasional papules, particularly on the forehead and cheeks. Several drugs induce acneiform lesions or make pre-existing acne worse, for example systemic steroids, phenytoin, isoniazid and lithium.

Oil-induced acne occurs when mineral oils come into close contact with the skin. This is often at unusual sites, such as the lower abdomen and thighs.

Chloracne is a specific change in which comedones appear after exposure to chlorinated chemical compounds. A famous example was the release of dioxin from the explosion at Seveso in Italy. Systemic upsets also occur.

Hidradenitis suppurativa

Although uncommon, this distinctive disorder results in very unpleasant chronic, relapsing sepsis in the apocrine areas of the axillae and groins (Fig. 6.7). Many apocrine glands open into the upper part of pilosebaceous follicles and comedonal occlusion of the ducts may be the initial event in hidradenitis.

Recurrent painful abscesses and sinus tracks develop. Many patients with hidradenitis have concurrent severe acne, or have suffered from acne in the past.

Some patients improve on long-term antibiotics, anti-androgens and/or isotretinoin acid, but many require plastic surgery.

Acneiform disorders

Several conditions mimic acne, but close examination will reveal important differences.

Pseudofolliculitis barbae (shaving rash): produces small papules in the beard area and is more common in those with naturally curly hair, especially Afro-Caribbeans. Occasionally small keloids develop. The process may involve the nape of the neck, when it is usually termed *acne keloidalis*. Treatment is unsatisfactory.

Acne excoriée (*des jeunes filles*) is typically seen in teenage girls who present with facial excoriations but very few primary lesions. There are no comedones. This is not true acne but a form of neurotic excoriation (see Chapter 20), and patients need to be given a clear explanation and helped to try and reduce the self-inflicted damage.

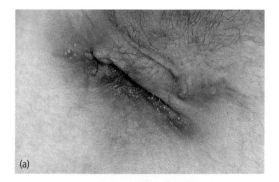

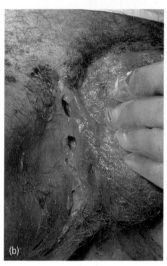

Figure 6.7 Hidradenitis suppurativa of (a) axilla; and (b) groin.

Pityrosporum folliculitis, caused by *Malassezia*, features follicular papules and pustules on the trunk, without other features of acne. The condition responds to antifungal agents such as miconazole.

In *keratosis pilaris*, small spiky projections develop at the mouth of hair follicles, especially on the upper, outer arms and shoulders. Lesions may appear on the face, especially in children, and are occasionally pustular. A family history is common. Topical retinoic acid may be helpful.

Rosacea is an important differential diagnosis of acne, and is sometimes called 'acne rosacea'. It occurs in both sexes, but most frequently affects middle-aged women. The sites of predilection are the central cheeks, forehead and glabellar region,

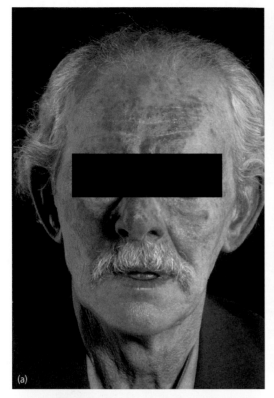

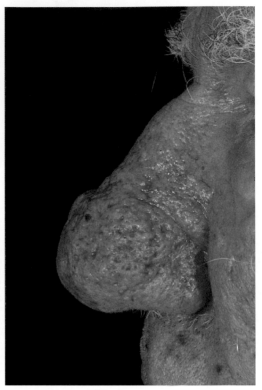

Figure 6.9 Rhinophyma.

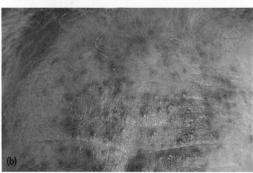

Figure 6.8 Rosacea (a) showing typical distribution; and (b) inflammatory papules and pustules.

end of the nose and chin (Fig. 6.8). The eruption consists of small papules and pustules arising in crops on an erythematous, telangiectatic background.

There are no comedones. Patients frequently complain that their face flushes easily with heat or alcohol, and migraines are more common. In men, severe involvement of the nose leads to marked sebaceous hyperplasia known as *rhinophyma* (Fig. 6.9).

The treatment of choice is tetracyclines, given for several weeks in similar doses to those for moderate acne (see above). Topical metronidazole is also effective and often used in combination with oral therapy. It may be possible to tail off the treatment, but the condition often recurs. Topical steroids make matters worse. Rhinophyma is best dealt with by plastic surgeons. Severe, resistant rosacea may respond to oral isotretinoin.

Perioral dermatitis (note for strict classical scholars: it should really be '*circum*-oral') produces a clinical appearance somewhat reminiscent of rosacea (see Fig. 22.3), and is often associated with topical steroid abuse. (For more details see Chapter 22.)

Chapter 7

Eczema

Introduction

The terms eczema (Greek, meaning 'to boil over') and dermatitis are synonymous. 'Atopic eczema' is therefore the same as 'atopic dermatitis', and 'seborrhoeic eczema' and 'seborrhoeic dermatitis' are the same. Eczema/dermatitis is a type of inflammatory reaction pattern in the skin which may be provoked by a number of external or internal factors.

Clinical features

The principal symptom of eczema is itching. The clinical signs depend on its aetiology, site and duration, but usually comprise erythema, oedema, papules, vesicles and exudation (Fig. 7.1). An acute eczema will have all these features, and might also have a bullous component. In a chronic eczema, oedema is not a prominent feature, but the epidermis becomes thickened and the skin surface markings are exaggerated (lichenification) (Fig. 7.2). A common feature of eczema of the hands or feet is the formation of painful fissures in the skin overlying joints.

A phenomenon which is seen with an acute dermatitis, particularly allergic contact dermatitis, is secondary spread of the eczema to sites distant from the originally affected area. Occasionally, most of the body surface is affected, and eczema is one cause of generalized exfoliative dermatitis.

Other changes in the skin which may accompany eczema include scratch marks and secondary bacterial infection. Prolonged scratching and rubbing the skin tends to polish fingernails, and patients with chronic eczema often have nails which look as if they have a coat of clear nail varnish.

Classification

We still have a great deal to learn about the aetiology of certain types of eczema, so any attempt at classification is based upon our present state of ignorance. A commonly employed system of classification divides cases of eczema into 'exogenous', where an external agent is responsible, and 'endogenous', where the problem is principally constitutional. There are, however, frequent cases in which more than one factor may be operating—for example, the hairdresser with hand dermatitis who suffers from atopic dermatitis and also has superimposed irritant dermatitis from contact with shampoos. Do not be too rigid in your attempts to classify a particular dermatitis—it may not fit a recognized category, and it might be preferable to use a more general term such as 'probably endogenous'. The following classification includes most of the types of eczema you are likely to encounter.

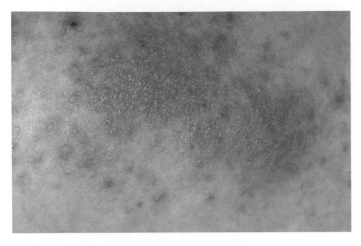

Figure 7.1 Typical eczema.

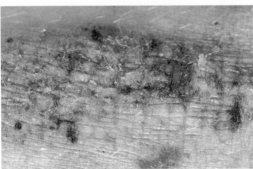

Figure 7.2 Lichenified eczema.

Eczema classification

Exogenous
- Primary irritant contact dermatitis
- Allergic contact dermatitis

Endogenous
- Atopic eczema
- Seborrhoeic dermatitis
- Discoid eczema
- Varicose eczema
- Endogenous eczema of the palms and soles
- Asteatotic eczema (eczema craquelé)

Exogenous eczema

Primary irritant dermatitis

Primary irritants physically damage the skin; they include acids, alkalis, detergents and petroleum products. Some strong irritants will produce an im-mediate effect, whereas with weaker irritants the effects are cumulative. Anyone suffering from atopic dermatitis is more susceptible to the effects of primary irritants. The housewife with a 'couch-potato' husband, eight children and no washing machine or dishwasher is a good candidate for a cumulative primary irritant dermatitis, because her hands will be perpetually immersed in wash-ing-up liquid and detergent. However, the wife of a merchant banker with 2.2 children, a nanny and a kitchen full of modern appliances is hardly likely to inconvenience her epidermis to the same de-gree. The typical appearance of housewives' hand dermatitis is dryness of the palms and fingertips, often with painful fissures in the skin creases and on the finger pulps.

Occupational irritant dermatitis is common. For example, hairdressing apprentices may spend a substantial part of the day with their hands im-mersed in shampoo on their clients' heads, and many develop irritant dermatitis. If they also have atopic eczema their hand problem often becomes so severe that they are forced to leave hairdressing. A similar situation is seen in machine-tool opera-tors whose hands are immersed in cutting fluid (Fig. 7.3). It follows that young people suffering from atopic dermatitis should be advised to avoid careers in occupations involving contact with irri-tants, such as hairdressing, engineering, vehicle mechanics, nursing and catering.

In theory, the treatment is simple—either re-move the patient from contact with the irritant, or

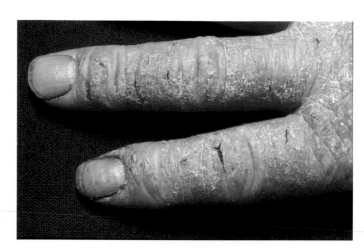

Figure 7.3 Hand dermatitis in a machine-tool operator.

protect the hands against it. In practice, it is often impossible to avoid contact with the irritant without changing jobs, and in many occupations the nature of the work means that wearing gloves is impracticable. The skin can be helped to a certain extent by the liberal use of emollients (see Chapter 22), but it cannot be restored to normal whilst exposure to irritants continues. What usually happens is that severe dermatitis eventually forces a change of occupation, or individuals with milder problems learn to tolerate them.

Allergic contact dermatitis

This is due to a delayed hypersensitivity reaction to an external allergen. There are innumerable chemicals that can act as allergens, but most rarely cause problems. Some chemicals are such potent allergens that a single exposure will cause sensitization, but many require multiple exposures before sensitization occurs. It is possible to be exposed to an allergen for years, and then suddenly develop hypersensitivity.

Frequent causes of contact dermatitis include nickel, colophony, rubber additives, chromate, hair dyes and topical medicaments—both their active ingredients and components of their bases.

Nickel dermatitis

Nickel is the most common cause of contact dermatitis in women, whereas contact allergy to nickel is uncommon in men. Sensitization to nickel usually occurs in childhood and early adult life as a result of ear piercing and the wearing of cheap costume jewellery. The problem usually begins with itchy earlobes, but it is dermatitis caused by the metallic components of other garments that brings the nickel-sensitive patient to the dermatologist. In the pre-miniskirt era, suspender dermatitis was the most common presentation of nickel sensitivity. Suspender belts were perhaps more functional than decorative in those days, and the bare metal clips produced patches of dermatitis on the thighs. With the advent of the miniskirt and tights, suspender dermatitis disappeared from the dermatology clinic. In more recent times, it is the jeans stud that has become an important source of nickel, and a patch of eczema adjacent to the umbilicus is virtually pathognomonic of nickel sensitivity (Fig. 7.4).

If nickel dermatitis is suspected, look at the skin on the earlobes and wrists. In spite of being aware that costume jewellery provokes a skin reaction, many women continue to wear a favourite pair of earrings from time to time, and will have dermatitis on the ears. Nickel dermatitis on the wrists is usually caused by the metal buckle on a watchstrap. Stainless steel in wrist-watches does not cause any problems because although steel contains nickel it is tightly bound and does not leach out.

The multitude of folk who have adopted the 'fashion' of having their delicate bodily parts

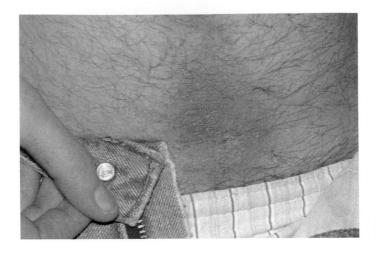

Figure 7.4 Contact dermatitis to nickel in jeans stud.

pierced are perhaps fortunate in that the various rings and barbells dangling and protruding from them are made of steel, and do not provoke dermatitis unless further embellished with costume jewellery. Anyone who is allergic to nickel should be advised to avoid costume jewellery (unless it is known to be nickel free), bare metal clips on underwear, metal buckles on shoes and metal zips. The metal stud on the front of jeans can be replaced by a button, and problems from watches can usually be avoided by wearing a 'Swatch' watch, as the only metal in contact with the skin is the stainless steel battery compartment.

Colophony

This is a resin which is a component of some adhesive plasters.

Rubber dermatitis

During the manufacture of rubber, chemicals are used to speed up the vulcanization process (accelerators) and to prevent its oxidation (antioxidants), and these can cause allergic contact dermatitis.

In recent years there has been a marked increase in the occurrence of reactions to natural rubber latex protein in latex gloves. Latex protein can pro-

voke an immediate hypersensitivity response, and reactions range from contact urticaria to rhinitis, asthma and anaphylaxis. Individuals affected are most often healthcare workers who frequently wear latex gloves, but patients who have undergone multiple procedures, most notably people suffering from spina bifida, may also be affected. A significant factor contributing to this problem appears to have been that the demand for latex gloves outstripped supply, and some manufacturers subsequently produced gloves containing large amounts of free latex protein. This situation has been remedied, and it is hoped that latex allergy will now become less of a problem.

Chromate

Chromium compounds have a number of industrial applications. They are also used in leather tanning, and are the major sensitizer in cement. Cement dermatitis is common in building workers.

Hair dye dermatitis

Contact sensitivity to hair dye usually presents as severe dermatitis affecting the face, ears and scalp margin. Hair dyes are also a cause of contact dermatitis on the hands of hairdressers. The chemical usually responsible for hair dye dermatitis, paraphenylenediamine (PPD), is also sometimes mixed with henna and used in temporary tattoos, a form of decoration which is quite popular at present, and this may be responsible for severe allergic contact dermatitis.

Topical medicaments

Medicament dermatitis is relatively common in dermatological practice, but perhaps not as common as might be expected if one considers the huge quantities of creams, lotions and potions used in the average household. Open any bathroom cabinet or bedside drawer in any house in the land and you will find creams for dry skin, creams for haemorrhoids, preparations for cuts and grazes, creams for insect bites and stings, and almost invariably a tube of a topical steroid.

Common causes of contact dermatitis in topical medicaments include antibiotics, particularly neomycin, local anaesthetics (except lidocaine (lignocaine), which is a rare sensitizer), antihistamines and preservatives. Dermatoses in which contact sensitivity to some of these agents may be a complicating factor include otitis externa, pruritus ani and venous leg ulcers. In recent years, contact allergy to topical steroids has emerged as a problem. It is usually discovered in patients who fail to respond or experience a deterioration in their skin condition whilst undergoing treatment with topical steroids.

Occupational contact dermatitis

If occupational factors are thought to be responsible for contact dermatitis, a detailed history, including precise information about the nature of an individual's work, is essential. This should include not only information about present occupation but also details of previous employment. A history of significant improvement of the dermatitis during holiday periods is typical of a work-related dermatosis. If someone tells you he was a 'saggar-maker's bottom knocker', enquire as to the nature of this exotic-sounding occupation (it used to be encountered in areas where ceramic ware was produced)—it is common to encounter terminolo-

gy which is specific to a certain occupation, and is incomprehensible to those outside the trade. Establish what materials are handled at work, and if there have been any changes which coincided with the onset of the dermatitis. It is also useful to know if any workmates have the same problem. Seeing a patient in the working environment is often important in determining the cause of a dermatitis.

Plant dermatitis

Plant dermatitis is relatively uncommon in the UK, but reactions to household plants usually involve *Primula obconica*. Garden plants can also cause problems, and in summer a combination of certain plants and sunlight can provoke a so-called *phytophotodermatitis*. Giant hogweed and other Umbelliferae are often implicated. A well-recognized scenario is the occurrence of a spattered blistering eruption in someone who, stripped to the waist in strong sunshine, has used a strimmer on weeds such as cow parsley (strimmer's dermatitis). In the USA, the most common cause of plant dermatitis is poison ivy. Dermatitis caused by plants tends to present with a linear, vesiculobullous reaction on the exposed parts of the body.

Diagnosis of allergic contact dermatitis

It is important to take a detailed history covering present occupation, previous occupations, hobbies and the use of topical medicaments. The distribution pattern of the dermatitis may suggest a possible allergen, and provoke further questions—for example, eczema adjacent to the umbilicus prompts enquiry about previous problems with earrings. Certain patterns are characteristic of a particular allergen: in the days when 'strike anywhere' matches were in common use, contact sensitivity to phosphorus sesquisulfide, which is present in the heads of the matches, was responsible for a combination of eczema on the face, in the ears, on the hands and on one or other thigh. The facial eczema was caused by contact with the smoke from the matches, the hand eczema by handling the matchbox, which had the chemical on the striking surface, and that on the thigh from carrying the box in a trouser pocket. The eczema in the ears was the result of using matches to clean them out!

However, when the cause is not as obvious, it may require considerable detective work to track it down, and patch testing (see Chapter 2) is an essential component of the investigative process. Patch testing is quite different from prick or scratch testing. It is a delayed hypersensitivity response, in which the reaction takes 48 h to develop, whereas prick or scratch tests elicit an immediate hypersensitivity response which develops within minutes. A standard battery of common allergens is used in routine patch testing, but other batteries of allergens, such as components of topical agents or occupational allergens, are also available. The majority of the allergens used are mixed in white soft paraffin to a specific concentration, because many are irritant in high concentration and might produce false-positive reactions. Patients sometimes claim that they are 'allergic' to materials they use at work, and these may be presented to the dermatologist, often in unmarked jars. Such materials are often irritants, and should not be used for patch testing without obtaining further information about their constituents and potential toxicity, otherwise they might bore an untidy hole in the patient's back.

Positive reactions must be interpreted in the context of the patient's presenting problem—not all positives will be relevant.

Wait until an acute eczema has settled before patch testing—positive reactions may exacerbate the eczema.

Treatment

Potent topical steroids (see Chapter 22) should be used to settle the eczema prior to patch testing. Once an allergen has been identified as the cause of a problem, the patient should be advised about its avoidance. If components of medicaments are involved, the patient's family doctor must be informed of what preparations the patient should avoid.

Endogenous eczema

Atopic eczema

The term 'atopy' implies a genetic predisposition to develop eczema, asthma and hay fever. A family history of atopy is common in patients with atopic eczema. However, a greater prevalence of atopic eczema in developed 'Westernized' countries than in underdeveloped countries, and evidence that the prevalence of atopic disease is increasing, are factors suggesting that environmental influences play a part in pathogenesis. Other factors in its complex pathogenesis are immunological abnormalities and emotional influences. Immunological abnormalities in the atopic state include increased serum total IgE and specific IgE antibody to ingested or inhaled antigens (such as house-dust mite allergens), and preferential activation of the Th2 subset of CD4+ T cells, which produce interleukin 4 (IL-4), IL-5 and IL-13, all of which are involved in regulation of IgE synthesis by B lymphocytes. Staphylococci colonize the skin of patients with atopic eczema, and staphylococcal exotoxins with superantigen properties are also thought to play a pathogenic role.

Atopic eczema is not present at birth, but frequently appears in the first year of life. In early childhood, the eczema is often generalized, but later a characteristic flexural involvement is seen—wrists, antecubital fossae, popliteal fossae and dorsa of feet (Fig. 7.5). The skin is dry and intensely itchy. As a result of constant scratching and rubbing, the affected areas become thickened (lichenification). The course is typically punctuated by episodic exacerbations.

Atopic eczema often resolves in childhood, but may persist into adolescence and adult life, and there is no way of predicting the outcome. Those whose skin has apparently reverted to normal remain susceptible to the effects of primary irritants, which may provoke a recrudescence of eczema.

The most common complication is secondary bacterial infection, producing folliculitis or impetigo. Viral warts and molluscum contagiosum occur more frequently in atopics, and herpes simplex

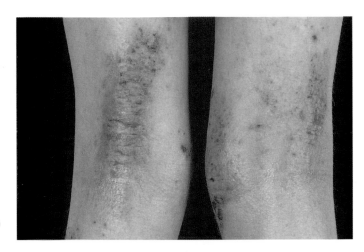

Figure 7.5 Flexural involvement in atopic eczema.

infection may lead to widespread skin lesions (see Chapter 3) and a severe illness (eczema herpeticum; Kaposi's varicelliform eruption).

Treatment

An important aspect of the management of a child with atopic eczema is sympathetic explanation of the nature of the condition to its parents.

Emollients are essential in the management of the dry skin in atopic eczema. There are numerous emollients available, and it is often necessary to try a number of preparations in order to find one that is suitable for a particular individual. They can be used in combination at bathtime—for example, one as a soap substitute, a bath oil in the water and an emollient cream afterwards.

Topical steroids are invaluable in the treatment of atopic eczema. In young children, mild steroids are the mainstay. In older children and adults, more potent steroids are required, but the aim should always be to use the weakest preparation sufficient to control the disease. A topical steroid/antibacterial combination may be useful if eczema frequently becomes secondarily infected— obvious secondary infection should be treated with a systemic antibiotic such as flucloxacillin or erythromycin. Emollient/antimicrobial combinations may also be useful in reducing bacterial colonization of the skin.

In recent years, topical preparations of the immunomodulators tacrolimus and pimecrolimus have become available for the treatment of atopic eczema. An advantage of these products is that, unlike topical steroids, they do not produce skin atrophy. At present, they are principally used in patients whose eczema has not responded to conventional therapy.

The wet-wrap technique is useful in the management of severe eczema, and medicated bandages such as zinc paste and ichthammol or zinc oxide and coal tar, applied over a topical steroid, are beneficial for eczema on the limbs. A sedative antihistamine at night may help to reduce scratching. Ultraviolet light treatment, either UVB or psoralens and UVA (PUVA therapy), helps some atopics, but the eczema often relapses when treatment is stopped. Ciclosporin (cyclosporin) may be of great benefit to patients with severe atopic eczema.

The value of dietary manipulation is controversial. Some children appear to be helped by elimination diets in which dairy products, food additives, nuts and other foods suspected of exacerbating eczema are excluded, but in many there is no obvious benefit. Most dermatologists reserve dietary manipulation for severely affected children who fail to benefit from other treatment methods. It is dangerous to manipulate a child's diet without expert advice, as this can lead to nutritional deficiencies.

Chinese herbal therapy is another controversial issue. Undoubtedly some individuals have benefited from Chinese herbal medicines, but there is concern about their potential for hepatotoxicity and nephrotoxicity, and some topical 'herbal' medicines have been shown to contain steroids.

Seborrhoeic dermatitis

This is a constitutional disorder whose exact pathogenesis is not fully understood, but in recent years the role of *Malassezia* yeasts has been emphasized.

Seborrhoeic dermatitis affects the scalp, face, presternal area, upper back and flexures. Scalp involvement presents as itchy, diffuse scaling on an erythematous background. On the face, there is scaly erythema in the nasolabial folds and on the forehead, eyebrows and beard area (Fig. 7.6). Lesions on the chest are often marginated. Flexural involvement produces a moist, glazed erythema. Particularly severe seborrhoeic dermatitis occurs in patients suffering from AIDS.

Seborrhoeic dermatitis usually requires treatment over many years, as there is no cure for this condition. It is important to make this clear to patients, who otherwise tend to try many treatments in their quest for a permanent solution to the problem. Topical hydrocortisone is effective, but the problem recurs when treatment is stopped. Steroid lotions or gels and tar shampoos will help the scalp. Ketoconazole shampoo and cream, and imidazole/hydrocortisone combinations, are also effective.

Discoid eczema

In this disorder, scattered, well-demarcated areas of exuding and crusting eczema develop on the trunk and limbs. A potent topical steroid is usually required to keep the condition controlled. Its aetiology is unknown.

Varicose eczema

Chronic venous hypertension is frequently associ-

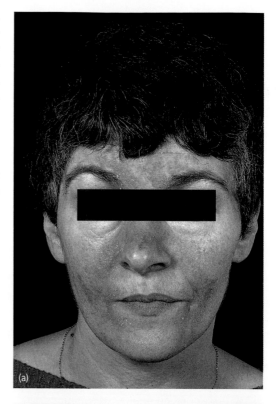

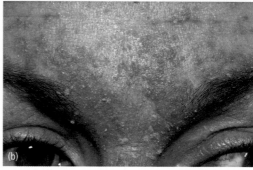

Figure 7.6 (a) and (b) Facial seborrhoeic dermatitis.

ated with eczematous changes on the legs. Secondary spread to the forearms may occur.

Mild or moderate potency topical steroids will usually suppress the eczema.

Endogenous eczema of the palms and soles

Some patients develop a symmetrical pattern of

eczema affecting the palms and soles which is chronic, and does not appear to be related to any external factors. Long-term treatment with potent topical steroids is usually required.

An episodic form of eczema of the palms and soles, in which bulla formation occurs, is known as *acute pompholyx* (Fig. 7.7). This develops rapidly, and can be severely incapacitating. Secondary bacterial infection is common. It usually responds to treatment with potassium permanganate soaks and a systemic antibiotic such as flucloxacillin or erythromycin. The trigger for these episodes is unknown.

Asteatotic eczema

With increasing age, the lipid content of the stratum corneum decreases, and elderly skin is particularly susceptible to 'degreasing' agents. Asteatotic eczema (also known as eczema craquelé) is usually seen on the legs, but it may also occur on the lower abdomen and arms, and occasionally it is generalized. It is common in elderly patients admitted to hospital and bathed more frequently than they bathe at home. A crazy-paving pattern develops (Fig. 7.8), and the skin itches. Treatment with an

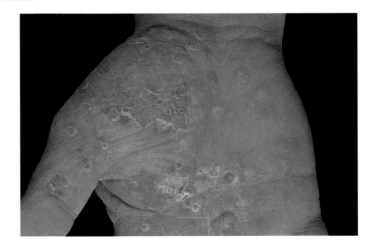

Figure 7.7 Pompholyx.

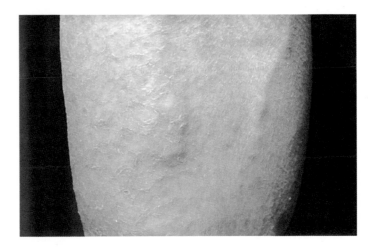

Figure 7.8 Eczema craquelé.

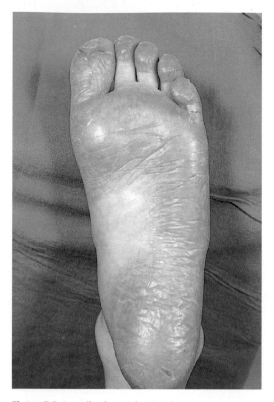

Figure 7.9 Juvenile plantar dermatosis.

emollient is sometimes adequate, but a mild topical steroid ointment is often necessary.

Juvenile plantar dermatosis

As its name suggests, this condition occurs in children. It is thought to be related to wearing training shoes and socks made of synthetic materials, and may represent a form of irritant dermatitis. It became prevalent in the 1970s when the 'trainer' was introduced as an item of footwear. The weight-bearing areas of the feet are dry and shiny, and painful fissures occur (Fig. 7.9). Changing to cotton or woollen socks and leather shoes sometimes helps, as does the liberal use of emollients. Topical steroids are usually ineffective. It almost invariably resolves by the early teens.

Chapter 8

Psoriasis

Dermatologists do it on a grand scale. (Anon)

Introduction

Psoriasis is one of the most common and most important of the inflammatory dermatoses: up to 3% of the population of Western countries, India and the Far East develop psoriasis during their lifetime. It is also common in parts of Africa. As most of those who develop psoriasis have lesions for the rest of their lives, it is clearly a considerable problem.

It is still not known why psoriasis develops when it does. There is undoubtedly a strong genetic component, particularly if the disease begins in youth or early adulthood. However, although a family history is common, there is often no clear-cut inheritance pattern. What does seem clear is that the cascade of changes described below probably result from an interaction between T cells and keratinocytes, with the involvement of various cytokines and chemoattractants—notably interleukins 1 and 8 (IL-1 and IL-8), tumour necrosis factor-alpha (TNF-α), E selectin and intercellular adhesion molecule-1 (ICAM-1).

Some well-recognized triggers may induce psoriasis in susceptible individuals, notably trauma and infections. Some authorities also maintain that stress may induce or exacerbate the condition. However, there is no clear understanding of what causes some areas of skin to turn into plaques of psoriasis while others remain normal.

Pathology

The pathological process is a combination of epidermal hyperproliferation and accumulation of inflammatory cells. The 'epidermal transit time' is markedly reduced from the normal 8–10 weeks to a few days. There is also increased vascularity of the upper dermis. Figure 8.1 provides a schematic representation of a psoriatic plaque. The cardinal features are given below.

Cardinal features

- Marked thickening of the epidermis (acanthosis)
- Absence of the granular cell layer
- Retention of nuclei in the horny layer (parakeratosis)
- Accumulations of polymorphs in the horny layer (microabscesses)
- Dilated capillary loops in the upper dermis

This basic picture, with some variations (e.g. increased size and number of polymorph abscesses in pustular psoriasis), unites all forms of psoriasis and the skin lesions of Reiter's syndrome.

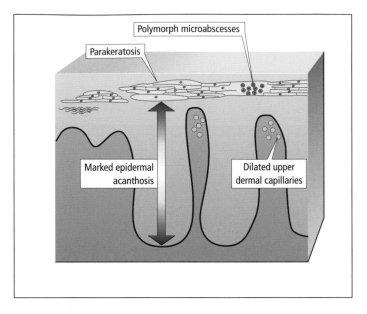

Figure 8.1 Schematic representation of a psoriatic plaque.

Clinical patterns of psoriasis

A number of different clinical patterns are recognized.

Some are common, others are rarer; some may be seen together or overlap. However, there is some merit in considering them separately.

Clinical patterns of psoriasis
• Classical plaque
• Scalp psoriasis
• Nail psoriasis
• Guttate
• Flexural
• 'Brittle'
• Erythrodermic
• Acute pustular
• Chronic palmo-plantar pustulosis
• Arthropathic psoriasis

Classical plaque psoriasis

This is the most common pattern. There are single or multiple red plaques, varying from a few millimetres to several centimetres in diameter, with a scaly surface (Fig. 8.2). If scraped very gently, the scale can be seen to reflect the light, giving a 'sil-very' effect (due to the parakeratotic horny layer). More vigorous rubbing induces capillary-point haemorrhage (Auspitz sign).

The plaques may develop on any part of the body, but psoriasis has a predilection for extensor surfaces: the knees, the elbows and the base of the spine. Lesions are often strikingly symmetrical. Involvement of the face is relatively uncommon. The scalp and nails are often affected (Figs 8.3 & 8.4), and an arthropathy may also occur.

Plaques tend to be chronic and stable, with little day-to-day change (as compared with 'brittle' psoriasis—see below). However, they may enlarge slowly, and may merge with adjacent areas. They may also resolve spontaneously. Occasionally, psoriatic plaques appear at the site of trauma or scarring. This is known as the Köbner or isomorphic phenomenon and is a characteristic, but not pathognomonic, feature. Exposure to UV radiation and natural sunlight often (but not always) improves psoriasis.

It is often said that psoriasis is not itchy, but in our experience a significant number of patients complain of severe itching, and most experience some itch at times. In fact, the Greek *psora* actually means itch. Some forms of psoriasis (e.g. guttate, flexural) are more prone to cause irritation.

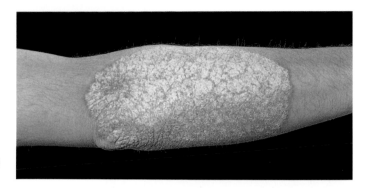

Figure 8.2 Psoriatic plaque on the elbow.

Scalp psoriasis

Scalp involvement is very common: indeed the scalp may be affected alone. It can be difficult to distinguish scalp psoriasis from severe seborrhoeic dermatitis (see also flexural psoriasis below), but psoriasis is generally thicker. As a rule of thumb, if you can feel scalp lesions as well as see them, they are probably psoriasis.

Lesions vary from one or two plaques to a sheet of thick scale covering the whole scalp surface (Fig. 8.3). Rarely, the scale becomes very thick and sticks in large chunks to bundles of hair. This is known as 'pityriasis amiantacea'. There may be temporary hair loss in severe scalp psoriasis.

Nail psoriasis

Nail abnormalities are frequent, and are important diagnostic clues if skin lesions are few, or atypical. Nail changes are almost always present in arthropathic psoriasis.

Two common findings may occur together or alone: pitting and onycholysis. Psoriatic nail pits are relatively large and irregularly arranged (Fig. 8.4), compared with those of alopecia areata. Onycholysis (lifting of the nail plate) starts as a red-brown area and progresses to separation of the nail plate from the nail bed (Fig 8.5). It is sometimes painful. These nail changes, particularly onycholysis, may also occur without other evidence of the disease.

Occasionally, pustular changes occur at the ends of the digits and in the nail bed (sometimes known

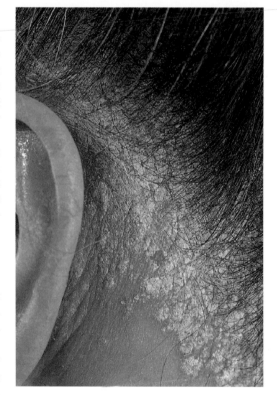

Figure 8.3 Scalp psoriasis.

as 'acrodermatitis continua'). Similar changes may accompany chronic palmo-plantar pustulosis (see below). In erythrodermic or pustular forms of psoriasis, the whole nail may become roughened and discoloured.

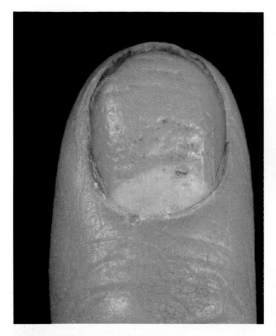

Figure 8.4 Nail pits in psoriasis.

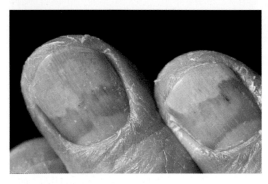

Figure 8.5 Psoriatic onycholysis.

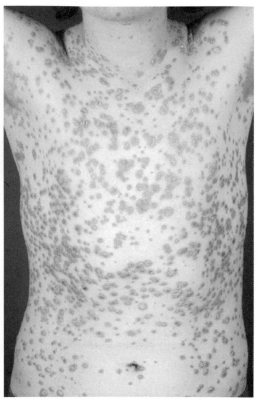

Figure 8.6 Guttate psoriasis.

Guttate psoriasis

Guttate psoriasis often develops suddenly, and may follow an infection, especially a streptococcal sore throat. It is a common way for psoriasis to present, particularly in young adults.

Gutta is the Latin for 'drop'. Most lesions are about a centimetre in diameter (Fig. 8.6), and usually paler in colour than established plaque psoriasis, at least initially. The main differential diagnosis is pityriasis rosea (see Chapter 15), best distinguished by the presence of parakeratotic scale in psoriasis, and the shape of the lesions (round in guttate psoriasis; oval in pityriasis rosea). Guttate psoriasis may itch.

The lesions of guttate psoriasis often resolve rapidly, but in some patients the patches enlarge and become stable plaques.

Flexural psoriasis

Flexural involvement in psoriasis may accompany typical plaque lesions, but is also commonly seen alone, or associated with scalp and nail changes. Lesions may occur in the groin, natal cleft, axillae, umbilicus and submammary folds. Maceration inevitably occurs, and the surface scale is often lost, leaving a rather beefy erythematous appearance (Fig. 8.7). It may be difficult to distinguish this from flexural seborrhoeic dermatitis, so look for nail changes or evidence of psoriasis elsewhere. Some dermatologists believe in an overlap state between the two, and call such changes 'sebo-psoriasis'.

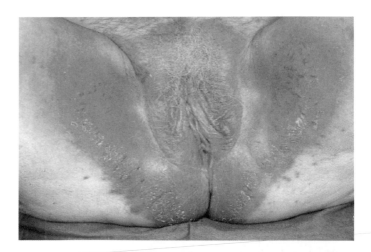

Figure 8.7 Flexural psoriasis.

Flexural psoriasis is often itchy. Watch out for a secondary contact sensitivity from the use of proprietary anti-itch preparations.

Brittle psoriasis

Occasionally you will see patients whose psoriasis does not consist of thick, stable plaques, but of thin, irritable scaly areas (Fig. 8.8). Lesions may arise *de novo* or develop suddenly in a patient whose psoriasis has been stable for years. One reason for this is systemic steroid therapy (often for another condition), and potent topical steroids can also induce stable psoriasis to become 'brittle'.

The significance of brittle psoriasis is that the lesions may rapidly generalize, especially if treated with potent agents (see treatment section below), leading to erythroderma (see Chapter 15) or even acute pustular psoriasis (see below).

Erythrodermic psoriasis

When psoriatic plaques merge to involve most or all of the skin, a state of erythroderma or exfoliative dermatitis results. The effects of this are discussed in Chapter 15.

Psoriasis may become erythrodermic by slow, inexorable progression, or very rapidly. Occasionally, erythrodermic psoriasis may appear *de novo*. Systemic steroids or potent topical steroids may precipitate this.

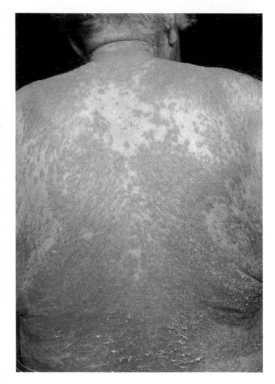

Figure 8.8 Widespread 'brittle' psoriasis.

Acute pustular psoriasis (of von Zumbusch)

This is a very serious condition. Patients with or without pre-existing psoriasis suddenly develop widespread erythema, superimposed on which are

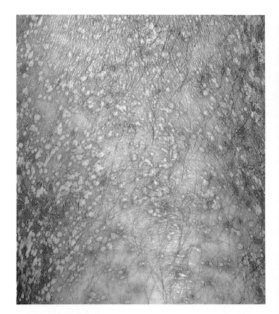

Figure 8.9 Acute pustular psoriasis.

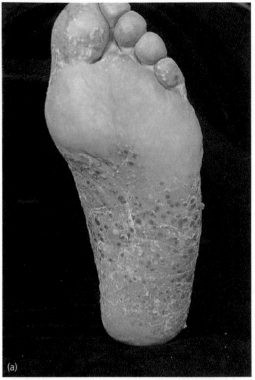

(a)

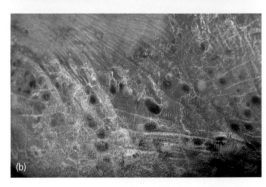

(b)

pustules. These may coalesce into lakes of pus (Fig. 8.9). The pustules are sterile.

The patient has a high, swinging fever and is toxic and unwell, with a leukocytosis. If the disease is unchecked, patients become increasingly ill and may die, often of secondary infections.

Chronic palmo-plantar pustulosis (pustular psoriasis of palms and soles)

There is some debate about the relationship between this condition and other forms of psoriasis. Biopsies reveal psoriasiform pathology, but it is unusual for patients to have chronic palmo-plantar pustulosis with other types of psoriasis.

The typical changes consist of erythematous patches with numerous pustules (Fig. 8.10). These gradually change into brown, scaly spots and peel off. The condition is usually uncomfortable or painful, rather than itchy.

Lesions may involve only a small area of one hand or foot, or cover the entire surface of both palms and soles. This may lead to considerable disability.

Figure 8.10 (a) Chronic palmo-plantar pustulosis. (b) The sterile pustules dry to form circumscribed brown areas that are later shed .

Treatment of psoriasis

The agents most widely used in the treatment of the skin lesions of psoriasis are:

Agents for treating psoriasis

Topical
- Emollients
- Tar
- Salicylic acid
- Topical steroids
- Dithranol (anthralin)
- Vitamin D analogues (e.g. calcipotriol, tacalcitol)
- Tazarotene
- Ultraviolet radiation

Systemic
- PUVA (psoralen + ultraviolet A)
- Retinoids
- Cytotoxics, e.g. methotrexate, azathioprine, hydroxy-carbamide (hydroxyurea)
- Systemic steroids
- Ciclosporin (cyclosporin)
- 'Biologicals': various monoclonal antibodies

It is an old adage that if there are many treatments for a disease, none works perfectly. This is certainly true of psoriasis. Although each modality is useful in some patients, all represent a compromise in terms of safety, effectiveness or convenience. Many patients require a regimen of different agents for different sites at different times.

Topical therapies

Many agents can be used topically to induce a remission or an improvement. Most are safe, but they are tedious for patients to use, as treatment may have to continue for months or, often, indefinitely.

Emollients

Some patients are prepared to tolerate plaques (especially on covered sites) if scaling can be controlled. Emollients such as white or yellow soft paraffin or lanolin may accomplish this.

Salicylic acid

Salicylic acid is a 'keratolytic' agent and helps to reduce scaling. It can be used with tar in mixtures, and is also combined with a potent topical steroid in commercially available preparations.

Tar

Tar has been used for many years, particularly in combination with UV radiation. The most effective preparations are extracts of crude coal tar. Attempts have been made to refine tar to make it more cosmetically acceptable, but the most effective forms still seem to be the darkest, smelliest and messiest. Consequently, not many patients will accept tar for widespread, routine use. However, in bath oils or in ointment mixtures, tar may be helpful, and it is very valuable in scalp disease.

Topical steroids

Topical steroids do not eradicate psoriasis, but may suppress it. Some dermatologists say they never use topical steroids in psoriasis because of the risks (they may induce 'brittle' psoriasis). However, if used with care in stable disease, and on the scalp and in the flexures, they can undoubtedly be useful.

Dithranol (anthralin)

Dithranol can convert psoriatic plaques into completely normal-looking skin. The mode of action is unknown. The 'Ingram regime'—a combination of dithranol, tar and UV radiation—has been used for years: most patients can be cleared in about 3 weeks of daily treatment. Originally, the dithranol was left on the skin for 24 h, but 'short-contact' therapy has been shown to be just as good.

Dithranol seems to work best in Lassar's paste (starch, zinc oxide and salicylic acid in white soft paraffin), but is also available in cream and ointment bases. Always begin with a low concentration (0.1%) and increase as necessary.

The main complications are staining (due to oxidation to a dye) and burning. Skin staining is temporary, but baths, bedding and clothes may be permanently marked. Dithranol burns can be very unpleasant, especially around the eyes and flexural areas. Patients must be taught to use dithranol carefully.

Vitamin D analogues and tazarotene

Vitamin D analogues (calcipotriol, tacalcitol, calcitriol) work well, and have rapidly found a place in routine management. They may irritate the face and in the flexures, and calcium levels may be disturbed if large quantities of vitamin D analogues are applied. Tazarotene is a retinoid and patients using it should avoid pregnancy because of theoretical teratogenicity.

Ultraviolet radiation

The use of UV therapy is well established, the most effective wavelengths being in the medium (UVB) range—and particularly 'narrow band' UVB. UVB must be used with care because it also induces sunburn. Patients require doses that *just* induce erythema but do not cause burning. The dose is then increased gradually. Treatment is usually given twice or thrice weekly until clearance is achieved. Adjunctive tar may make UVB more effective.

UVB is theoretically carcinogenic (as is tar), but surprisingly few psoriasis sufferers develop skin cancers.

Systemic therapies

Psoralen + ultraviolet A (PUVA)

Psoralens form chemical bonds with DNA in the presence of UV radiation. The patient is given one of these agents (8-methoxypsoralen and trioxsalen are the most common), either used as a soak or taken by mouth 2h before exposure to long-wavelength UV light (UVA), initially twice weekly. Protective glasses are worn to prevent ocular damage. There is a significant long-term risk of keratoses and epithelial cancers with PUVA.

Cytotoxic drugs

The most effective and widely used cytotoxic is methotrexate, a folic acid antagonist. Most psoriasis responds to a *once weekly* dose of 7.5–20 mg. Other drugs include azathioprine and hydroxycarbamide (hydroxyurea).

All cytotoxics have unwanted effects, particularly bone marrow suppression. This is rare with methotrexate, but may occur in an idiosyncratic manner unrelated to dose. The major problem with methotrexate is hepatotoxicity, particularly fibrosis, with chronic use. Alcohol appears to exacerbate this tendency. Patients require regular and continuous monitoring of liver function and it is now considered best practice to measure the levels of a circulating collagen precursor (PIIINP). A sustained high level indicates the need for a liver biopsy. Methotrexate also inhibits spermatogenesis and is teratogenic. Its use is therefore restricted to severely affected patients.

Retinoids

Vitamin A derivatives help some patients with psoriasis. The most commonly used is acitretin. Retinoids have a number of side-effects, including dry lips, nose-bleeds, hair loss, hyperlipidaemia, liver function test abnormalities and teratogenicity.

Systemic steroids

In very severe psoriasis, steroids may occasionally be necessary, but should not be used alone.

Ciclosporin (cyclosporin)

This immunosuppressive drug works extremely well, even in very severe psoriasis. It is nephrotoxic and very expensive.

Biologicals (monoclonal antibodies)

A number of agents have been developed, aimed at specific compounds, such as TNF-α, involved in immuno-inflammatory diseases such as rheumatoid arthritis and psoriasis. Examples include infliximab, etanercept and efalizumab. These are expensive and require administration by injection under controlled conditions.

Treatment of clinical patterns of psoriasis

The choice of therapeutic regimen in psoriasis is dictated by the type and extent of lesions, and by the effects on the patient's quality of life. A balance will often have to be struck between the need for improvement and the inconvenience and/or side-effects of the agent(s) concerned.

Chronic plaque psoriasis

Dithranol is a theoretical first choice, but the patient's lifestyle, or side-effects, may make it impractical. If so, vitamin D analogues or topical steroids (with or without tar and salicylic acid) are often used. UV radiation may help. If lesions become very extensive, or if there are serious psychosocial problems, PUVA, retinoids, cytotoxic drugs or biologicals may be indicated.

Scalp psoriasis

Tar shampoos are helpful, but will seldom control thick plaques alone. Tar gels may help, but the best topical remedy is Unguentum Cocois Co.—a mixture including tar and salicylic acid. This is massaged in at night and washed out the following morning. Topical steroid lotions, with or without salicylic acid, are also used.

Nail psoriasis

Nail changes do not respond to topical treatment, and systemic drugs are seldom justified for nails alone.

Guttate psoriasis

This is most effectively treated with UV radiation together with emollients and a tar-based ointment. If patients cannot find time to attend for treatment, a combination of moderately potent topical steroids and vitamin D analogues may be the best option.

Flexural psoriasis

Psoriasis in the flexures poses problems. Mild tar/corticosteroid mixtures may be effective, but long-term use of topical steroids can cause striae. Dithranol, used in very low concentrations, can be successful, but burning is common and underclothes are stained. UVB and PUVA generally fail to reach the affected areas. Vitamin D analogues help, but can sting. Tacrolimus and pimecrolimus have been used recently (and for facial lesions).

Brittle psoriasis

Brittle psoriasis requires careful management. Avoid potent topical steroids, strong tar and salicylic acid preparations. Emollients or very dilute steroids may bring the skin into a more stable condition, but PUVA, retinoids or methotrexate may be needed, at least for a short time.

Erythrodermic and acute pustular psoriasis

Although both of these states may settle with conservative management, it is more likely that systemic treatment will be required. Such intervention can be life saving. The most common choice is methotrexate, but ciclosporin also works well. When the condition is stable, the dose should be gradually reduced and the drug stopped if possible. However, many patients relapse and require long-term treatment. Biologicals may become an important option in such patients.

Chronic palmo-plantar pustulosis

Nothing really works well in this condition. Tar pastes, potent topical steroids or dithranol are often ineffective. Vitamin D analogues may be worth a try, as is oral acitretin, and PUVA to the hands and feet may provide control, but relapse is common with any therapy.

Arthropathic psoriasis

One of the most unpleasant complications of psoriasis is arthropathy, affecting up to 10% of psoriatics. There are four basic patterns.

Psoriatic arthropathy patterns

- Distal interphalangeal joint involvement
- Seronegative rheumatoid-like joint changes
- Large joint mono- or polyarthropathy
- Spondylitis

Most commonly the distal interphalangeal joints are involved, with the other changes listed above in descending order of frequency. Psoriatic arthropathy is erosive and may result in joint destruction.

Psoriatics who develop the spondylitic form are usually HLA B27 positive, and there is some overlap between psoriatic arthropathy and other seronegative arthritides.

Non-steroidal anti-inflammatory drugs and methotrexate are used. Biologicals are gaining increasing importance in this group of patients.

Reiter's syndrome

This disorder, which frequently follows a diarrhoeal illness or non-specific urethritis in HLA B27-positive individuals, is discussed in Chapter 19. Occasionally skin lesions known as 'keratoderma blennorrhagicum' develop. Palmar and plantar lesions may become very gross (Fig. 8.11), and lesions elsewhere are clinically very similar to psoriasis. Histologically, keratoderma blennorrhagicum is indistinguishable from psoriasis.

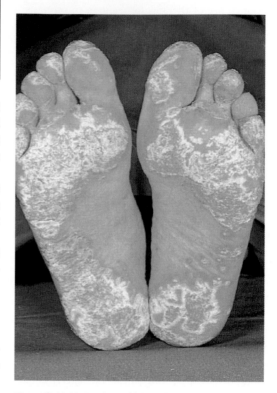

Figure 8.11 Keratoderma blennorrhagicum.

Chapter 9

Benign and malignant skin tumours

Know ye not that a little leaven leaveneth the whole lump? St Paul (1 Corinthians, 5:6)

Introduction; classification of skin tumours

Lumps on or in the skin are extremely common and the workload associated with them is rising because:

1 The age of the population as a whole is increasing (many skin tumours are more common in elderly people).
2 Skin cancer is increasing in all age groups.
3 There is increasing public awareness of the importance of skin tumours.

Most skin tumours are benign, often representing only a cosmetic nuisance. However, it is important to distinguish these from malignant or potentially malignant tumours quickly and effectively, as decisions about what should be done about a lesion can only be made after a diagnosis to this minimum level has been made.

The skin is a complex organ system, with both benign and malignant tumours described for every component. Table 9.1 presents a simplified version of the wide variety of skin tumours.

General treatment principles for skin tumours

It is worth reviewing briefly the techniques used to treat skin tumours. This will avoid repetition.

The first important principle is that, unless the diagnosis is certain, some tissue should be preserved for histology. Failure to do this will mean missed malignancies, and is one explanation for patients who present with mysterious lymphatic or distant deposits from unknown primary sites.

Surgical removal or biopsy

These techniques have already been described and illustrated (see Figs 2.2 & 2.3). Removal of small skin tumours is quick, simple and economical. If the tumour is too large for primary excision, take a small incisional biopsy, remembering to cross the edge from normal to abnormal tissue. There is no evidence that such a biopsy adversely affects the outcome, although it is advisable to avoid incisional biopsy of suspected invasive melanomas if possible (see below).

Curettage and/or cautery ('C&C')

This is a perfectly satisfactory method for the removal of superficial tumours.

Table 9.1 Tumours, benign or malignant, found in the epidermis and dermis.

Types of tumours	Types of tumours
A: Epidermis (for naevi see Chapter 10)	**C: Dermis (for naevi see Chapter 10)**
Benign	*Benign*
• Seborrhoeic keratosis	• Fibrous tissue:
• Skin tags	dermatofibroma
• Keratoacanthoma	• 'Neural' tissue, e.g. neurofibroma
• Viral warts (see Chapter 3)	• Vascular tissue:
• Clear cell acanthoma	angioma/angiokeratoma
• Tumours of skin appendages, e.g. sweat glands,	pyogenic granuloma
sebaceous glands, hair follicles	glomus tumour
• Epidermal cysts	
	Dysplastic/malignant
Dysplastic/malignant	• Fibrosarcoma
• Basal cell carcinoma	• Neurofibrosarcoma
• Actinic (solar) keratosis	• Angiosarcoma, including Kaposi's sarcoma
• Squamous cell carcinoma:	
in situ (Bowen's disease)	**D: Pseudo-tumours**
invasive	• Chondrodermatitis nodularis helicis
• Paget's disease	• Hypertrophic and keloid scars
• Tumours of skin appendages	
	E: Lymphomas
B: Melanocytes (for naevi see Chapter 10)	• Cutaneous T-cell lymphoma (mycosis fungoides)
Benign	• Cutaneous B-cell lymphoma
• Freckle and lentigo	
	F: Extension from deeper tissues
Dysplastic/malignant	
• Dysplastic naevus (see Chapter 10)	**G: Metastatic deposits**
• Lentigo maligna	
• Malignant melanoma:	
lentigo maligna melanoma	
superficial spreading	
nodular	
acral	

C&C

1 Use a curette (Volkmann spoon) to scrape off lesions
2 Touch the raw base a few times with cautery or a hyfrecator* to control oozing
3 Apply a simple dressing and/or antiseptic

*A hyfrecator produces electrical haemostasis and desiccation.

Pedunculated tumours can be removed by slicing with cautery across the base.

Cryotherapy

The use of cryotherapy for tumours has become very popular. It is ideal for superficial skin tumours because it is quick and leaves relatively little scarring. However, histological interpretation of cryo-biopsies is not easy and it should be used only if: the tumour is definitely benign; or an incisional biopsy has already been performed. Cryotherapy is not appropriate for melanomas. The best agent is liquid nitrogen.

Cryotherapy

1 Apply nitrogen with cotton-wool buds, or by specially designed spray or probe instruments
2 Wait until a halo of frozen skin 1 mm around the tumour is obtained
3 Maintain halo for 10 s for benign, 30 s for malignant tumours
4 Allow to thaw, and repeat (two 'freeze/thaw cycles')

The patient should be told to expect blistering, followed by healing with crust formation. The lesion should separate within 3 weeks.

Radiotherapy

Radiotherapy is an effective treatment method for basal and squamous cell carcinomas, and may be the most practical option for very large tumours in elderly patients. However, it is not ideal for the trunk and limbs, and the choice between excision and radiotherapy should be based on individual circumstances.

Radiotherapy can also control secondary tumour deposits.

Lasers and photodynamic therapy

There is an increasing interest in the application of laser technology to treating skin disease, especially for skin tumours and naevi (see Chapter 10), but also for hirsutism (see Chapter 13), scars, wrinkles and other 'defects'. Many benign epithelial tumours will respond to ablation by a CO_2 laser but are also very easily treated by other, simpler and cheaper means. Pigmented lesions respond to several lasers, but their place has yet to be fully established.

Photodynamic therapy (PDT) is a process involving the use of a porphyrin and light, which destroys superficial lesions such as Bowen's disease and superficial basal cell carcinomas.

Specific tumours

We shall first consider benign tumours, and then dysplastic and malignant processes, discussing the most common and most important of these.

Some skin lumps are hamartomatous malformations. Such a lesion in the skin is termed a 'naevus'. Naevi are discussed separately in Chapter 10.

Benign tumours—epidermal

Seborrhoeic keratoses (seborrhoeic warts; basal cell papillomas)

You are bound to see seborrhoeic keratoses, if only in passing while examining a chest. They are most frequent in elderly people, and may be solitary or multiple. Occasionally there are hundreds of lesions (a tendency which may be familial).

Clinical features. A flat-topped area of skin with a 'stuck-on' appearance (Fig. 9.1). They may be pale, but are often pigmented, sometimes deeply so. The surface is often said to be greasy, but a more useful sign is the granular look occasioned by small surface pits and irregularities.

Sites of predilection. Head and neck; backs of hands and forearms; trunk.

Differential diagnosis. Usually straightforward, but darkly pigmented lesions can be mistaken for melanomas. On the face, seborrhoeic keratoses may remain virtually flat, causing difficulty in distinguishing them from senile lentigo or lentigo maligna (see below). Another diagnostic problem arises if lesions become inflamed. There may be crusting and bleeding, and biopsy for histology may be necessary.

Treatment. If deemed necessary (there is no malignant potential), the best approach for smaller lesions is cryotherapy. Larger ones may be better treated by curettage and cautery or excision.

Skin tags (acrochordons)

Many people develop these small pedunculated lesions around the neck and in the axillae. Increasing age and obesity are predisposing factors.

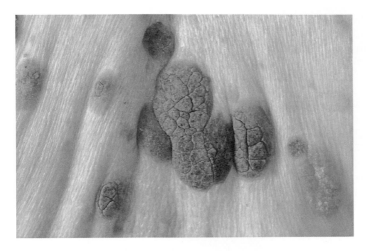

Figure 9.1 Typical seborrhoeic warts.

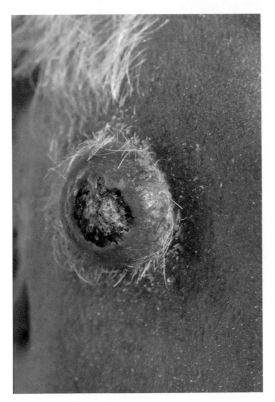

Figure 9.2 Keratoacanthoma.

Differential diagnosis. Small melanocytic naevi may look similar, and so may small pedunculated seborrhoeic keratoses.

Treatment. They can be removed very easily by snip and cautery/hyfrecation.

Keratoacanthoma (once called 'molluscum sebaceum')

This tumour is an oddity. Some authors classify keratoacanthoma as malignant because the histology resembles a squamous cell carcinoma (see below). Keratoacanthomas are much more common in elderly people.

Clinical features. Lesions arise rapidly, reaching a maximal size over the course of 6–8 weeks (Fig. 9.2). The tumour is round, with rolled edges and a central keratin plug. The base is often red and inflamed, and may be painful. Ultimately, the tumour begins to shrink, often almost as quickly as it enlarged, and disappears completely, leaving a small puckered scar.

Sites of predilection. Almost invariably on light-exposed skin.

Differential diagnosis. Differentiation from basal cell carcinoma (see below) can be made on the basis of the history of rapid growth and on the perfect roundness of the lesion.

The main problem is to distinguish *prospectively* between a keratoacanthoma and a squamous cell carcinoma. By definition a keratoacanthoma should resolve spontaneously, but this cannot be determined in advance. Incisional biopsies may not help because of the close similarities to squamous cell carcinoma.

Treatment. It is reasonable to wait expectantly for a short while if a lesion is very typical, especially in elderly or frail patients. However, if there is any diagnostic doubt, keratoacanthomas are best removed and sent for histology. There is a case for removing such a lesion early, in order to avoid the necessity for a more complex procedure if it becomes much larger.

Other benign epidermal tumours

Viral warts are discussed in Chapter 3, and the other benign epidermal tumours listed are rare.

Epidermal cysts

There are three common forms of epidermal cyst—pilar, epidermoid and milium.
1 Common scalp cysts are correctly termed 'pilar' or 'trichilemmal' cysts. There may be several, and a familial predisposition is usual.
2 Epidermoid cysts may be found anywhere, but are most common on the head, neck and trunk. They often follow severe acne; there is a cystic swelling within the skin, usually with an overlying punctum.

Treatment. Both types can be removed easily under local anaesthetic using a linear incision over the surface.
3 Milia are extremely common keratin cysts, which may occur spontaneously or after trauma or blistering. In some families, there is an inherited tendency to develop clusters on the cheeks and around the eyes (Fig. 9.3).

Treatment. Milia can be treated by incision, pricking out or cautery/hyfrecation.

Benign melanocytic tumours

Freckles (ephelides) and lentigines

Freckles are areas of skin containing melanocytes, normal in number but hyper-responsive to UV radiation. They are genetically determined: we all know typical freckly red-heads.

Lentigines are flat pigmented areas composed of increased numbers of melanocytes.

Melanocytic naevi are discussed in Chapter 10.

Benign tumours—dermal

Dermatofibroma

Dermatofibromas (Fig. 9.4) are made up of fibrous tissue and some blood vessels. It is not

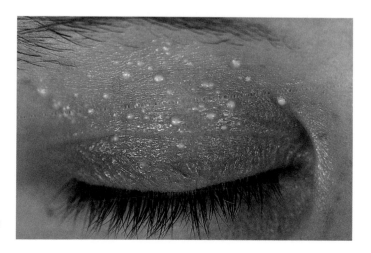

Figure 9.3 Milia around the eyes: a characteristic site.

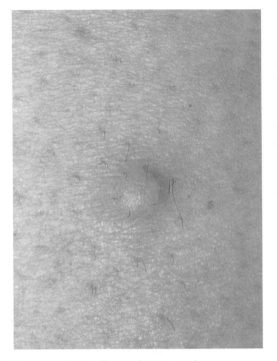

Figure 9.4 Dermatofibroma (histiocytoma).

known why they occur, but they may follow minor trauma.

Clinical features. More common in women; often easier to diagnose by touch than by sight—they feel like small lentils.

Sites of predilection. Limbs; legs more than arms.

Differential diagnosis. Occasionally, heavy pigmentation can cause confusion with melanoma.

Treatment. Excision may be cosmetically indicated.

Angioma

Angiomas are collections of aberrant blood vessels within the dermis and/or subcutaneous tissues. Some are developmental defects, commonly present at birth, and these are discussed in Chapter 10. Others develop during adult life, such as the ubiquitous Campbell de Morgan spot (Fig. 9.5).

Pyogenic granuloma

Pyogenic granulomas are benign reactive inflammatory masses composed of blood vessels and fibroblasts.

Clinical features. They erupt rapidly, usually have a polypoid appearance (Fig. 9.6) and a 'collar' around the base; profuse contact bleeding is common.

Sites of predilection. Sites of an injury or infection, often on a digit.

Differential diagnosis. They must be differentiated from squamous cell carcinomas and amelanotic melanomas.

Treatment. Removal by curettage or excision should always be followed by histological examination.

Others

You may encounter several other benign dermal or subcutaneous lumps: neurofibromas, for example in von Recklinghausen's neurofibromatosis (see Chapter 11); various benign fibroblastic tumours; and lipomas, which are readily identified by their soft texture and lobulated outline.

If there is any doubt about any dermal or subcutaneous lump, it is best removed for histology.

Pseudo-tumours

Chondrodermatitis nodularis helicis (painful nodule of the ear)

This curious lesion is not a tumour, but an inflammatory process.

Clinical features. A small umbilicated nodule on the rim of the ear, usually in men (Fig. 9.7); the clue is that it is painful, especially in bed at night.

Differential diagnosis. It is often confused with basal cell carcinomas or other tumours.

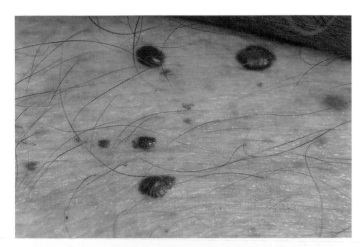

Figure 9.5 Campbell de Morgan spots.

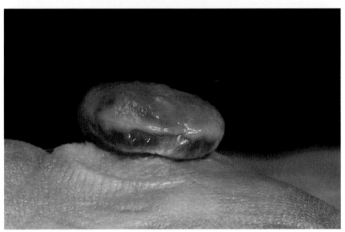

Figure 9.6 Side view of a typical pyogenic granuloma.

Treatment. Cryotherapy may work or it can easily be excised.

Hypertrophic scars and keloids

Scar formation can be very exuberant, especially at some sites (see below) and in children, young adults and black skin. A hypertrophic scar flattens after about 2 years, whereas a keloid persists and spreads laterally beyond the original site (keloids can become very large).

Clinical features. Protuberant masses usually following cuts, ear-piercing, burns, acne and BCG inoculations (if performed high on the shoulder); some appear to develop spontaneously; keloids often itch.

Sites of predilection. Chest, upper back, shoulder, pubic region, ear lobes.

Differential diagnosis. Any soft-tissue tumour, especially if there is no preceding history of trauma.

Treatment. Excision generally leads to recurrence, and management can be extremely difficult. Intralesional steroids, cryotherapy and radiotherapy before and after excision all have their advocates.

Dysplastic and malignant tumours

The term 'dysplasia' implies that the skin has been partly, or wholly, replaced by cells with neoplastic features. When this results in invasion of adjacent

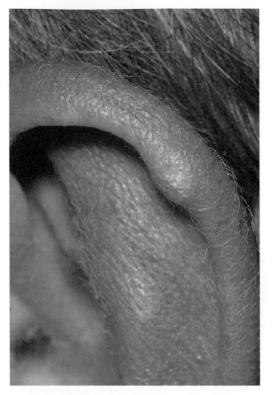

Figure 9.7 Chondrodermatitis nodularis helicis.

tissue, the process can genuinely be said to be 'malignant'.

Cutaneous dysplasias and malignancies are increasingly common, especially in ageing skin and in skin exposed to prolonged UV radiation. Other factors are also associated with dysplastic skin changes:

1 Most forms of ionizing radiation (UV light, X-rays, γ-rays) are powerful inducers of skin cancer.

2 There are a number of known carcinogens, such as: exposure to some industrial oils, tars and bitumen; exposure to soot used to result in scrotal cancers in chimney sweeps.

3 Skin cancers are a feature of some genetic diseases: a notable example is xeroderma pigmentosum, in which the repair of UV-induced DNA damage is faulty.

4 Skin cancers occur more commonly in immunosuppressed individuals following renal and cardiac transplantation.

Dysplastic/malignant epidermal tumours

Basal cell carcinoma (BCC)

The most common malignant skin tumour is often known as a 'rodent ulcer'.

Clinical features. Most begin as a nodule (Fig. 9.8) which spreads slowly outwards, usually leaving a central depression (creating the classical 'rolled edge'); usually skin is coloured with a translucent look (often described as 'pearly'); telangiectatic vessels on the surface are very characteristic, and account for the frequent presenting complaint of contact bleeding; metastasis is extremely rare, but local invasion can be destructive (Fig. 9.9) and BCCs can spread along bony passages into the skull.

Variants. Several distinctive clinical variants of the BCC are recognized (see below).

Sites of predilection. Predominantly the face, but BCCs occur on other sun-exposed sites, in the hair-bearing scalp, behind the ear and on the trunk (where the superficial pattern is common).

Differential diagnosis. Early lesions may be confused with naevi; superficial BCCs are often treated as inflammatory; heavy pigmentation may suggest a melanoma; morphoeic tumours can be very difficult to diagnose.

Clinical variants of BCC

Morphoeic A flat growth pattern which results in a scar-like appearance; it can be very difficult to know where the tumour begins and ends, and local invasion is more common

Superficial Lesions grow for many years and may be many centimetres across; usually solitary; multiple tumours may indicate previous arsenic ingestion; characteristically, a 'worm-like' edge is seen (Fig. 9.10)

Pigmented Pigmentation is usually patchy but may be very dark and dense

---

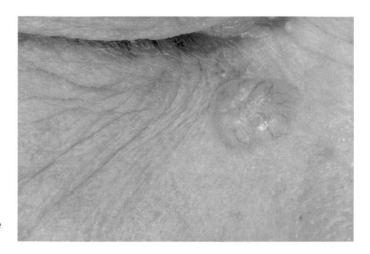

Figure 9.8 Basal cell carcinoma. Note the telangiectatic vessels.

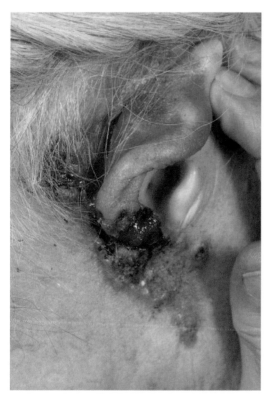

Figure 9.9 Basal cell carcinoma. Such destruction gives rise to the term 'rodent ulcer'.

Treatment. Excision, biopsy and radiotherapy or, for superficial tumours, curettage, cryotherapy or photodynamic therapy; careful assessment of morphoeic tumours is needed—a technique known as 'microscopically controlled surgery' (Mohs surgery) may be helpful; it is particularly important to deal adequately with lesions around the eyes, nose and ears. The use of topical therapies for superficial types, notably imiquimod (a promoter of interferon-alpha), has been pioneered more recently.

Actinic or solar keratoses

These are areas of dysplastic squamous epithelium without invasion, but actinic keratoses do have low-grade malignant potential and their presence indicates unstable epithelium.

Clinical features. Red and scaly patches (Fig. 9.11) which characteristically wax and wane with time; many hundreds of lesions may occur in heavily sun-exposed individuals.

Sites of predilection. Light-exposed skin, especially the face, forearms, dorsa of hands, lower legs and bald scalp.

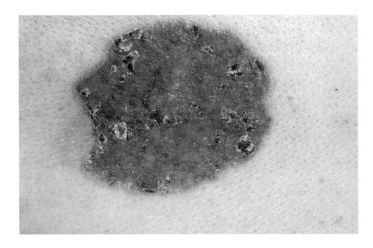

Figure 9.10 Superficial basal cell carcinoma.

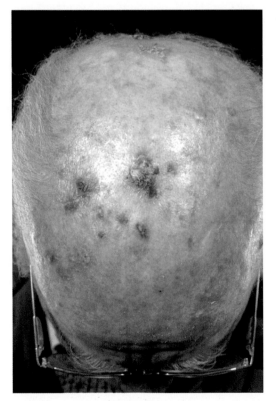

Figure 9.11 Multiple solar keratoses.

Differential diagnosis. Lesions of chronic discoid lupus erythematosus can be difficult to distinguish, and some are pigmented, leading to confusion with lentigo maligna (see below).

Treatment. Cryotherapy is best for small numbers of lesions; large areas on the face and scalp can be treated with the topical agents diclofenac sodium and 5-fluorouracil; in very elderly patients it may be best to do nothing.

Squamous cell carcinoma (SCC) *in situ* (or Bowen's disease)

Bowen's disease is an SCC confined to the epidermis, and is common below the knees in elderly women. Invasive change does occur but is rare.

Clinical features. Usually a solitary patch of red scaly skin, although multiple areas may occur; Bowen's disease is asymptomatic.

Variant. Erythroplasia of Queyrat—non-invasive dysplastic changes may also occur on the penis, where the clinical appearance is of a velvety red plaque. Although given a separate name, it is essentially the same as Bowen's disease elsewhere.

Sites of predilection. Light-exposed skin; may occur on non-exposed areas such as the trunk.

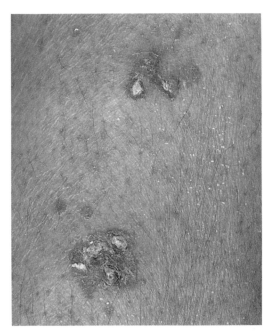

Figure 9.12 Two patches of Bowen's disease.

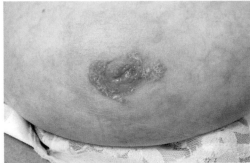

Figure 9.13 Paget's disease of the nipple.

Differential diagnosis. There is a superficial resemblance to psoriasis (Fig. 9.12), but the surface scale is adherent rather than flaky. Removal of scale leaves a glistening red surface that does not bleed. As arsenic was used in the past to treat psoriasis, keep an eye out for Bowen's disease in elderly psoriasis sufferers.

Similar changes on one nipple should always suggest the possibility of *Paget's disease* (Fig. 9.13); a biopsy should be performed as there is always an underlying breast carcinoma.

Treatment. Should be treated by excision, curettage, cryotherapy or photodynamic therapy; very large areas may require radiotherapy.

Invasive squamous cell carcinoma

SCCs are locally invasive, and may metastasize to regional lymph nodes and beyond (especially lip, mouth and genital lesions). UV radiation is important aetiologically, but other factors also play a role: smoking in lip and mouth cancers; wart virus in genital lesions.

Clinical features. These may be very varied, typically either:
1 a keratotic lump,
2 a rapidly growing polypoid mass (Fig. 9.14) or
3 a cutaneous ulcer.
SCCs are often surrounded by actinic keratoses.

Sites of predilection. Sun-exposed sites; SCCs also develop on the lips (Fig. 9.15), in the mouth and on the genitalia.

Differential diagnosis. Keratotic lesions may closely resemble hypertrophic actinic keratoses.

Treatment. Biopsy of any suspicious lesion; definitive treatment is by surgical removal or radiotherapy.

Dysplastic/malignant melanocytic tumours

Lentigo maligna (or Hutchinson's malignant freckle)

The term 'lentigo maligna' describes a patch of malignant melanocytes, in sun-damaged skin, which proliferate radially along the dermoepidermal junction and deep around hair follicles, often for many years. An invasive component may develop at any time.

Clinical features. A flat, brown area with irregular pigmentation.

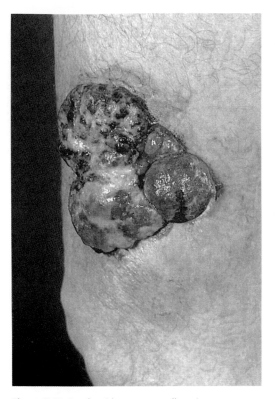

Figure 9.14 A polypoid squamous cell carcinoma.

Sites of predilection. Almost always on the face (Fig. 9.16).

Differential diagnosis. Can be difficult to distinguish from flat seborrhoeic keratoses, pigmented actinic keratoses and simple lentigines.

Treatment. Biopsy is essential; definitive treatment is a matter of debate; excision is our preferred option because of the risk of recurrences with cryotherapy or topical therapies; in very elderly patients it may be reasonable to do nothing and follow the patient carefully.

Malignant melanoma patterns

Lentigo maligna melanoma
The appearance of a nodule of invasive melanoma within a lentigo maligna.

Superficial spreading melanoma (SSM)
The most common in the UK; the tumour has a radial growth phase before true invasion begins
- Clinical features:
  irregularly pigmented brown/black patch with an irregular edge (Fig. 9.17)
  may itch or give rise to mild discomfort
  may bleed
- Sites of predilection:
  most frequently on the leg in women and the trunk in men, but may occur anywhere
- Differential diagnosis:
  naevi in the young
  flat seborrhoeic keratoses in older patients

Nodular melanoma
The tumour exhibits an invasive growth pattern from the outset
- Clinical features:
  rapidly growing lumps (Fig. 9.18)
  occasionally warty (verrucous melanoma) or non-pigmented (amelanotic melanoma)
- Sites of predilection:
  may occur anywhere
- Differential diagnosis:
  other rapidly growing tumours

Acral melanoma
Rare in the UK, but much more common in other countries (e.g. Japan); it is virtually the only type of melanoma seen in Asian or Afro-Caribbean patients
- Clinical features:
  a pigmented patch on the sole or palm or an area of subungual pigmentation
- Differential diagnosis:
  can be confused with a viral wart
  must be distinguished from haematoma
Some MMs arise in pre-existing melanocytic naevi, although estimates of the frequency of this vary from 5% to over 50%.

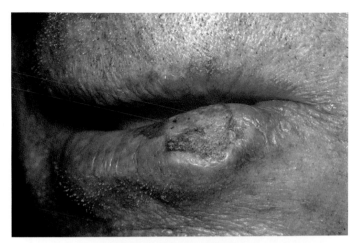

Figure 9.15 Squamous cell carcinoma on the lip.

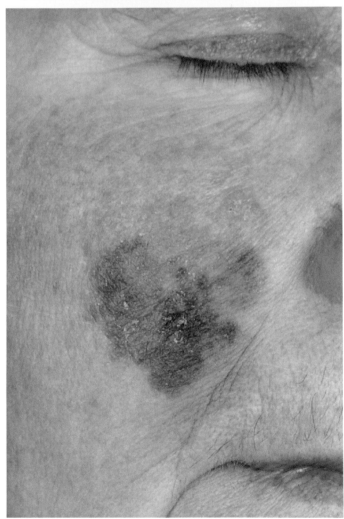

Figure 9.16 Lentigo maligna.

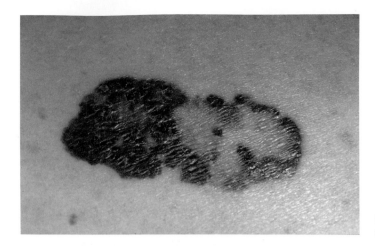

Figure 9.17 Superficial spreading melanoma.

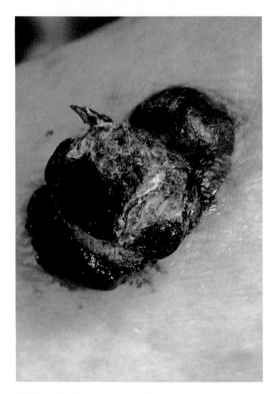

Figure 9.18 Large nodular melanoma.

Malignant melanoma (MM)

This is the most dangerous of the malignant skin tumours. Melanomas, other than lentigo maligna melanoma, occur in a relatively younger age group than other skin cancers. The incidence is rising rapidly, even in temperate climates, probably as a result of the increase in intermittent sun exposure that is now so fashionable. Rising standards of living have permitted more sunny holidays abroad (and at home), during which the most important 'activity' is sunbathing.

Periods of exposure to very strong sunlight with sunburn are particularly risky and there is evidence that childhood sun exposure may be important. Some melanomas arise in pre-existing melanocytic naevi (see Chapter 10). It seems that the incidence of this varies from country to country.

There are four recognized patterns of malignant melanoma (see box on page 92).

Treatment of malignant melanoma

The prognosis in MM is related to the depth of tumour invasion at first excision, regardless of the original type. It is standard practice to measure invasion using a technique known as the 'Breslow thickness' (Fig. 9.19). If the tumour is less than 1.5 mm at first excision, 5-year survival is about 90%; if the depth is over 3.5 mm this falls to 40% or less.

All types of melanoma should therefore be excised at the earliest possible opportunity. Radiotherapy and chemotherapy have little to offer at present in curing the disease. There is some debate about how wide the excision margins should be, but they are becoming narrower. There is certainly no harm in initial narrow excision. The

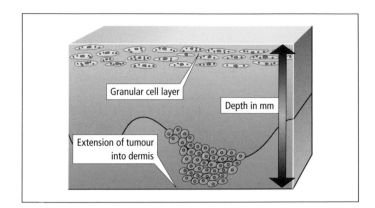

Figure 9.19 Breslow thickness.

urgency is to remove the melanoma—further procedures can be considered later.

In acral melanoma it may be necessary to perform a confirmatory biopsy before definitive treatment, which may involve amputation.

Encouraging early presentation

The most effective way of improving treatment is to increase public awareness of MMs and thereby prompt people to seek advice about suspicious lesions. Many doctors now use a checklist (see box).

Prevention of epithelial and melanocytic malignancies

Both types of epithelial skin cancers, and melanomas, are more common in those who burn easily in the sun: those with fair skin, fair or red hair and blue or green eyes (skin types I and II—see Chapter 12). Melanomas are also more common in individuals with many melanocytic naevi.

It is logical therefore to recommend that those at risk avoid excessive sun exposure:
1 No one should allow themselves to be sunburnt.
2 It is best to avoid midday sun (between 11 a.m. and 3 p.m.) or, at least, wear adequate clothing and hats.
3 Sun-screens offering a high degree of protection should be used.

Those who tan easily and those with brown or black skin need not take such draconian precautions, but for all children sun exposure should be restricted.

Malignant melanoma checklist

• Is an existing mole getting larger or a new one growing? After puberty, moles usually do not grow. (This sign essentially refers to adults, remember that naevi may grow rapidly in children (see Chapter 10).)
• Does the lesion have an irregular outline? Ordinary moles are a smooth, regular shape
• Is the lesion irregularly pigmented? Particularly, is there a mixture of shades of brown and black?
• Is the lesion larger than 1 cm in diameter?
• Is the lesion inflamed or is there a reddish edge?
• Is the lesion bleeding, oozing or crusting?
• Does the lesion itch or hurt?

Any pigmented lesion, whether newly arising or already present, which exhibits three or more of the seven listed features, and especially one of the first three, should be treated as highly suspicious.

Dermal malignant tumours

Malignant sarcomas may develop in the skin.

Clinical features. Indolent, slow-growing nodules, which become fixed to deeper tissues.

Differential diagnosis. Difficult to categorize without biopsy.

Treatment. Wide excision is generally required; in one tumour of this kind (*dermatofibrosarcoma protuberans*), very wide indeed.

Kaposi's sarcoma

This malignant vascular tumour merits special mention in spite of its rarity. 'Classical' Kaposi's sarcoma occurs in Ashkenazi Jews and northern Italians. A much more aggressive form is seen in Africans and in people with AIDS.

Clinical features. Purplish plaques and nodules.

Sites of predilection. Legs in the classical form; anywhere in the aggressive form.

Differential diagnosis. Other vascular lesions.

Treatment. Biopsy; symptomatic treatment with radiotherapy.

Lymphomas

Lymphomatous involvement of the skin may be secondary, for example in non-Hodgkin's B-cell lymphoma. However, the skin may be the original site, especially in cutaneous T-cell lymphoma (often called 'mycosis fungoides').

Clinical features. Variable; some areas remain unchanged or grow slowly for years; red, well-circumscribed, scaly plaques and tumours eventually develop (Fig. 9.20).

Differential diagnosis. Lesions can be confused with eczema or psoriasis.

Treatment. Biopsy is essential but can be difficult to interpret. DNA phenotyping of cells may be of value; definitive treatment varies with the stage, but includes radiotherapy, PUVA and chemotherapy.

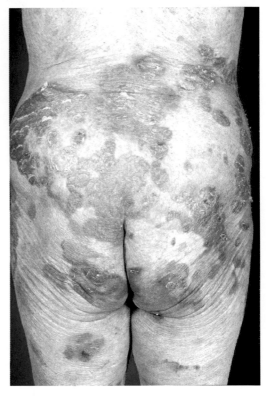

Figure 9.20 Areas of mycosis fungoides (cutaneous T-cell lymphoma).

Extension from deeper tissues and metastases

Tumours of underlying structures, such as breast, may invade the skin. The skin may also be the site of metastatic deposits from internal cancers such as bronchogenic carcinoma (see Chapter 19).

Chapter 10

Naevi

Ten thousand saw I at a glance (Wordsworth)

Introduction

Naevi are extremely common—virtually everyone has some. However, the word 'naevus' can give rise to confusion. Much of the difficulty is due to the term being used in several different ways, in addition to that outlined below. Some writers use the word without qualification for the most common cutaneous hamartoma, the melanocytic naevus (see below). The word is also applied to lesions that are not congenital at all, such as the 'spider naevus' (which is probably better called 'spider telangiectasis'). This is complicated further by some true 'naevi' being called 'moles' or 'birthmarks'. Thus, a lump described as a 'mole' may be a melanocytic naevus, but may also be any small skin lesion, especially if pigmented, while 'birthmark' is accurate enough as far as it goes, but many naevi develop after birth.

We use the word 'naevus' to mean a cutaneous hamartoma (a lesion in which normal tissue components are present in abnormal quantities or patterns). This encompasses 'naevi' which are not actually present at birth, because the cells from which they arise are.

Any component of the skin may produce a naevus, and they may be classified accordingly (Table 10.1). We need only discuss the most important: epithelial and organoid naevi, vascular naevi and melanocytic naevi.

Epithelial and 'organoid' naevi

These are relatively uncommon developmental defects of epidermal structures: the epidermis itself, hair follicles, and sebaceous glands. There are two important types, the epidermal naevus and the sebaceous naevus.

Epidermal naevus

Circumscribed areas of epidermal thickening may be present at birth or develop during childhood; many are linear. Very rarely, there are associated central nervous system (CNS) abnormalities.

Becker's naevus presents as a pigmented patch first seen at or around puberty, usually on the upper trunk or shoulder, and which gradually enlarges and frequently also becomes increasingly hairy.

Sebaceous naevus

Sebaceous naevi are easily overlooked at birth. They begin as flat, yellow areas on the head and neck which, in the hairy scalp, may cause localized alopecia. Later, the naevus becomes thickened and warty, and basal cell carcinomas may arise within it. These naevi are best excised during adolescence.

Melanocytic naevi

The most common naevi are formed from

Table 10.1 A classification of naevi.

Naevi classification
Epithelial and 'organoid'
• Epidermal naevus
• Sebaceous naevus
• Hair follicle naevus
Melanocytic
Congenital
• Congenital melanocytic naevus
• Mongolian blue spot
Acquired
• Junctional/compound/intradermal naevus
• Sutton's halo naevus
• Dysplastic naevus
• Spitz naevus
• Blue naevus
Vascular
Telangiectatic
• Superficial capillary naevus
• Deep capillary naevus
• Rare telangiectatic disorders
Angiomatous
Other tissues
• Connective tissue
• Mast cell
• Fat

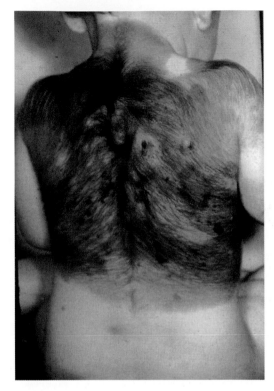

Figure 10.1 Giant congenital melanocytic naevus.

melanocytes that have failed to mature or migrate properly during embryonic development. We all have some. Look at your own skin or, better, that of an attractive classmate, to see typical examples!

It is convenient to categorize melanocytic naevi by clinical and histopathological features, because there are relevant differences (Table 10.1). The first is whether they are present at birth (congenital) or arise later (acquired).

Congenital

Congenital melanocytic naevus

One per cent of children have a melanocytic naevus at birth.

These vary from a few millimetres to many centimetres in diameter. There is a rare, but huge and grossly disfiguring variant, the 'giant' congenital melanocytic or 'bathing trunk' naevus (Fig. 10.1).

Small to medium congenital melanocytic naevi may be slightly more prone to develop melanomas than acquired lesions, but the giant type definitely predispose to melanoma development. Prepubertal malignant melanoma is extremely rare, but nearly always involves a congenital naevus. This leads to a paradox: small, low-risk naevi are easily removed but larger lesions with higher malignant potential require extensive, even mutilating, surgery. Each case must be judged on its own merits, and decisions must involve the parents/carers and the child.

Mongolian blue spot

Most children of Mongoloid extraction and many South Asian and Afro-Caribbean babies are born with a diffuse blue-black patch on the lower back and buttocks. There are melanocytes widely dispersed in the dermis (the depth is responsible for the colour). The area fades as the child grows, but may persist indefinitely. Unwary doctors have mistaken Mongolian blue spots for bruising, and accused parents of baby-battering.

Acquired

Acquired melanocytic naevus

A melanocytic naevus is 'acquired' if it develops during postnatal life, a phenomenon that is so common as to be 'normal'. Most only represent a minor nuisance, and 'beauty spots' were once highly fashionable.

The first thing to understand is that each naevus has its own life history. This will make the terms applied to the different stages in their evolution clearer (Fig. 10.2).

The lesion (Fig. 10.3) is first noticed when immature melanocytes proliferate at the dermoepidermal junction (hence 'junctional'). After a variable period of radial growth, some cells migrate vertically into the dermis ('compound'). Eventually the junctional element disappears and all melanocytic cells are within the dermis ('intradermal'). Different melanocytic naevi will be at different stages of development in the same individual.

Most melanocytic naevi appear in the first 20 years of life, but may continue to develop well into the forties. They are initially pigmented, often heavily and even alarmingly, but later may become pale, especially when intradermal. Most disappear altogether: very few octogenarians have many.

Their importance (apart from cosmetic) is 3-fold:
• some malignant melanomas develop in a pre-existing naevus (the chance of this happening in any one lesion is infinitesimally small);
• the possession of large numbers of acquired melanocytic naevi is a risk factor for melanoma;
• melanocytic naevi can be confused with melanomas.

Any melanocytic lesion which behaves oddly should be excised for histology, but remember that, by definition, all melanocytic naevi grow at some stage. Therefore, growth alone is not necessarily sinister, especially in younger individuals.

Most naevi undergoing malignant change show features outlined in Chapter 9; but . . . 'if in doubt, lop it out'!

There are several variants of the acquired melanocytic naevus (see below).

Acquired melanocytic naevus

Sutton's halo naevus A white ring develops around an otherwise typical melanocytic naevus; the lesion may become red and disappear (Fig. 10.4). This is an immune response of no sinister significance and unknown cause

Dysplastic naevus Some lesions look unusual and/or have unusual histopathological features; this may affect just one or two naevi, but some people have many; such individuals may be part of a pedigree in which there is a striking increase in melanoma ('dysplastic naevus syndrome')

Blue naevus The characteristic slate-blue colour (Fig. 10.5) is due to deep dermal melanocytes; they are most common on the extremities, head and buttocks

Spitz naevus Sometimes called juvenile melanoma ± the prefix 'benign'; benign lesion of children which has a characteristic brick-red colour; Spitz naevi can be confused histologically with malignant melanoma

---

Vascular naevi

Vascular blemishes are common. Some present relatively minor problems, whereas others are very disfiguring. The terminology used for these lesions can be confusing and is by no means uniform. We have adopted what we consider to be a simple and practical approach based on clinical and pathological features.

Vascular malformations

Superficial capillary naevus

These pink, flat areas, composed of dilated capillaries in the superficial dermis (Fig. 10.6), are found in at least 50% of neonates. The most common sites are the nape of the neck ('salmon patches' or 'stork marks'), the forehead and glabellar region ('stork marks' again), and the eyelids ('angel's kisses'). Most facial lesions fade quite quickly, but those on the neck persist, although often hidden by hair.

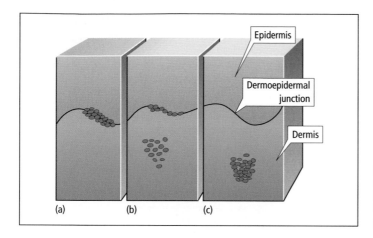

Figure 10.2 The phases of the acquired melanocytic naevus: (a) junctional; (b) compound; (c) intradermal. These stages are part of a continuum, and each lasts a variable time.

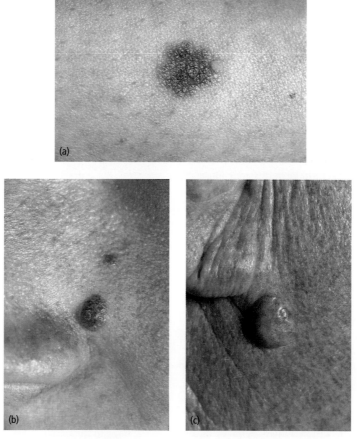

Figure 10.3 The development phases of an acquired melanocytic naevus: (a) junctional (flat, pigmented); (b) compound (raised, pigmented); (c) intradermal (raised, no pigment).

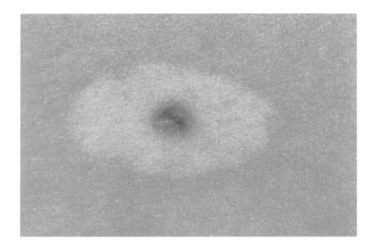

Figure 10.4 Sutton's 'halo' naevus.

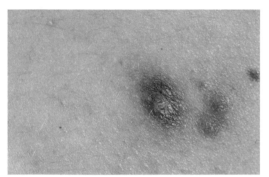

Figure 10.5 Blue naevus.

Deep capillary naevus

'Port-wine stains' or 'port-wine marks' are formed by capillaries in the upper and deeper dermis. There may also be deeper components and these may gradually extend over time.

Deep capillary naevi are less common but more cosmetically disfiguring than superficial lesions. Most occur on the head and neck and are usually unilateral, often appearing in the territory of one or more branches of the trigeminal nerve (Fig. 10.7). They may be small or very extensive.

At birth, the colour may vary from pale pink to deep purple, but these malformations show no tendency to fade. Indeed they often darken with time, and become progressively thickened. Lumpy, angiomatous nodules may develop.

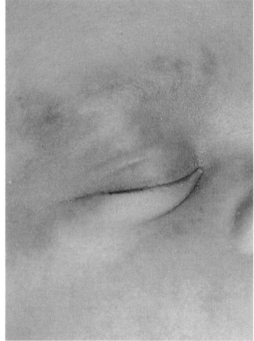

Figure 10.6 Superficial capillary naevus.

These lesions are most unattractive, and patients often seek help. Modern lasers can produce reasonable results, and a range of cosmetics can be used as camouflage.

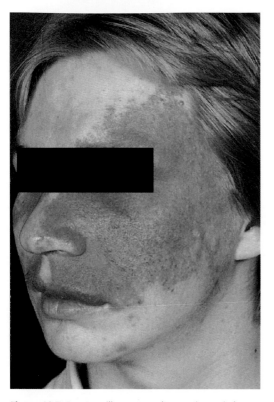

Figure 10.7 Deep capillary naevus ('port-wine stain').

There are three important complications.

Complications of deep capillary naevus

• An associated intracranial vascular malformation may result in fits, long-tract signs and mental retardation. This is the Sturge–Weber syndrome
• Congenital glaucoma may occur when lesions involve the area of the ophthalmic division of the trigeminal nerve
• Growth of underlying tissues may be abnormal, resulting in hypertrophy of whole limbs—haemangiectatic hypertrophy

---

If a deep capillary naevus is relatively pale, it may be difficult to distinguish from the superficial type, especially in the neonatal period. It is therefore wise always to give a guarded initial prognosis and await events.

Childhood angiomas

These are quite distinct from pure vascular malformations in that they are characterized by the presence of actively growing and dividing vascular tissue, but some lesions are genuinely mixtures of malformation and angioma. Terminology can be difficult: 'strawberry naevus' and 'cavernous haemangioma' are still terms in common use, but we prefer simply to call them childhood or infantile angiomas.

The majority arise in the immediate postnatal period, but some are actually present at birth. They may appear anywhere, but have a predilection for the head and neck and the napkin area (Fig. 10.8). Most are solitary, but occasionally there are more, or there are adjacent/confluent areas (and are called 'segmental' by some authorities). Lesions usually grow rapidly to produce dome-shaped, red-purple extrusions which may bleed if traumatized. The majority reach a maximum size within a few months. They may be large and unsightly.

Spontaneous resolution is the norm, sometimes beginning with central necrosis, which can look alarming. As a rule of thumb, 50% have resolved by the age of 5 and 70% by age 7. Some only regress partially, and a few require plastic surgical intervention.

The management, in all but a minority, is expectant. It is useful to show parents a series of pictures of previous patients in whom the lesion has resolved

Specific indications for intervention:
1 If breathing or feeding is obstructed.
2 If the tumour occludes an eye—this will lead to blindness (amblyopia).
3 If severe bleeding occurs.
4 If the tumour remains large and unsightly after the age of 10.

Treatment of complications 1–3 is initially with high-dose prednisolone, which may produce marked shrinkage. If this fails, and with persistent tumours, complex surgical intervention may be required.

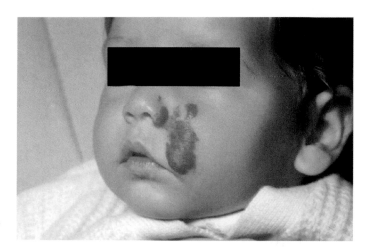

Figure 10.8 Cavernous haemangioma on the face.

Rare angiomatous naevi

Rarely, infants are born with multiple angiomas of the skin and internal organs. This is known as *neonatal or miliary angiomatosis* and the prognosis is often poor.

Other naevi

Naevi may develop from other skin elements, including connective tissue, mast cells and fat. For example, the cutaneous stigmata of tuberous sclerosis are connective tissue naevi (see Chapter 11), and the lesions of urticaria pigmentosa are mast cell naevi.

Chapter 11

Inherited disorders

There is only one more beautiful thing than a fine healthy skin, and that is a rare skin disease. (Sir Erasmus Wilson, 1809–84)

A number of skin conditions are known to be inherited. Many are rare, and will therefore only be mentioned briefly. There have been major advances in medical genetics in recent years, and the genes responsible for many disorders have been identified and their roles in disease clarified.

Several diseases in which genetic factors play an important part, such as atopic eczema, psoriasis, acne vulgaris and male-pattern balding, are described elsewhere in the book.

The ichthyoses

The term ichthyosis is derived from the Greek *ichthys*, meaning fish, as the skin has been likened to fish scales. The ichthyoses are disorders of keratinization in which the skin is extremely dry and scaly (Fig. 11.1). In the majority of cases, the disease is inherited, but occasionally ichthyosis may be an acquired phenomenon, for example in association with a lymphoma. There are several types of ichthyosis, which have different modes of inheritance (Table 11.1).

Autosomal dominant ichthyosis (ichthyosis vulgaris)

This is the most common, and is often quite mild.

The scaling usually appears during early childhood. The skin on the trunk and extensor aspects of the limbs is dry and flaky, but the limb flexures are often spared. Ichthyosis vulgaris is frequently associated with an atopic constitution.

The principal abnormality is reduced production of profilaggrin—this is the precursor of filaggrin, which is a major component of keratohyalin granules.

X-linked recessive ichthyosis

This type of ichthyosis only affects males. The scales are larger and darker than those of dominant ichthyosis, and usually the trunk and limbs are extensively involved, including the flexures. Corneal opacities may occur, but these do not interfere with vision. Affected individuals are deficient in the enzyme steroid sulfatase—the result of abnormalities in its coding gene. The majority of patients have complete deletion of the steroid sulfatase gene, located on the short arm of the X chromosome at Xp 22.3.

Both X-linked ichthyosis and autosomal dominant ichthyosis improve during the summer months.

Ichthyosiform erythroderma and lamellar ichthyosis

A non-bullous form of ichthyosiform erythro-

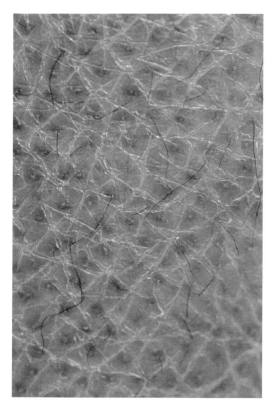

Figure 11.1 Ichthyosis.

Table 11.1 The ichthyoses.

Primary (congenital) ichthyosis
Ichthyosis vulgaris (autosomal dominant ichthyosis)
X-linked recessive ichthyosis
Non-bullous ichthyosiform erythroderma
Bullous ichthyosiform erythroderma (epidermolytic hyperkeratosis)
Netherton's syndrome
Sjögren–Larsson syndrome
Refsum's disease

Acquired ichthyosis
Lymphoma
AIDS
Malnutrition
Renal failure
Sarcoidosis
Leprosy

---

derma (NBIE) is recessively inherited and is usually manifest at birth as a 'collodion baby' appearance (see below). Thereafter there is extensive scaling and redness. Lamellar ichthyosis is also recessively inherited, and affected infants also present as collodion babies. Scaling is thicker and darker than in NBIE and there is less background erythema. These conditions are probably parts of a clinical spectrum caused by several different genes.

In bullous ichthyosiform erythroderma (epidermolytic hyperkeratosis), which is dominantly inherited, there is blistering in childhood and later increasing scaling until the latter predominates. There is a genetic defect of keratin synthesis involving keratins 1 and 10.

The ichthyosiform erythrodermas are all rare, as are some other ichthyosiform disorders, including Netherton's syndrome (ichthyosis linearis circumflexa and bamboo hair), Sjögren–Larsson syndrome (ichthyosis and spastic paraparesis) and Refsum's disease (ichthyosis, retinitis pigmentosa, ataxia and sensorimotor polyneuropathy).

Acquired ichthyosis

When ichthyosis develops in adult life, it may be a manifestation of a number of diseases, including underlying lymphoma, AIDS, malnutrition, renal failure, sarcoidosis and leprosy.

Treatment

Treatment consists of regular use of emollients and bath oils. Urea-containing creams are also helpful. Oral retinoid treatment may be of benefit in the more severe congenital ichthyoses.

Collodion baby

This term is applied to babies born encased in a transparent rigid membrane resembling collodion (Fig. 11.2). (Collodion is a solution of nitrocellulose in alcohol and ether used to produce a protective film/membrane on the skin after its volatile components have evaporated, and also employed as a vehicle for certain medicaments.) The

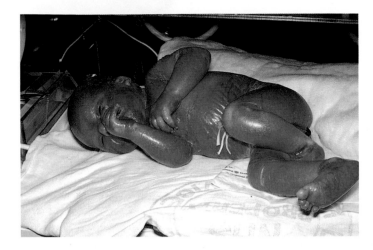

Figure 11.2 Collodion baby.

membrane cracks and peels off after a few days. Some affected babies have an underlying ichthyotic disorder, whereas in others the underlying skin is normal. Collodion babies have increased transepidermal water loss, and it is important that they are nursed in a high humidity environment and given additional fluids.

Palmo-plantar keratoderma

Several rare disorders are associated with massive thickening of the horny layer of the palms and soles. The most common type is dominantly inherited. Many medical texts mention an association of palmo-plantar keratoderma (tylosis) with carcinoma of the oesophagus—in fact this is extremely rare.

Darier's disease (keratosis follicularis)

This is a dominantly inherited disorder which is usually first evident in late childhood or adolescence. It is caused by mutation in the *ATP2A2* gene at chromosome 12q24.1, which encodes an enzyme important in maintaining calcium concentrations in the endoplasmic reticulum. The abnormality results in impaired cell adhesion and abnormal keratinization.

The characteristic lesions of Darier's disease are brown follicular keratotic papules, grouped together over the face and neck, the centre of the chest and back, the axillae and the groins (Fig. 11.3). The nails typically show longitudinal pink or white bands, with V-shaped notches at the free edges (Fig. 11.4). There are usually numerous wart-like lesions on the hands (acrokeratosis verruciformis).

It is exacerbated by excessive exposure to sunlight, and extensive herpes simplex infection (Kaposi's varicelliform eruption) can occur.

Darier's disease responds to treatment with retinoids.

Epidermolysis bullosa

This group of hereditary blistering diseases is described in Chapter 14.

Ehlers–Danlos syndrome

There are a number of distinct variants of this condition, all of which are associated with abnormalities of collagen, principally defective production. The most common are dominantly inherited, but all types of Ehlers–Danlos syndrome are rare. Typical features are skin hyperextensibility and fragility, and joint hypermobility. In certain types, there is a risk of rupture of major blood vessels because of deficient collagen in the vessel wall.

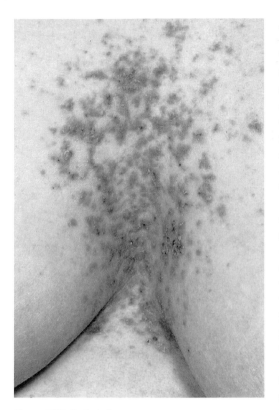

Figure 11.3 Darier's disease.

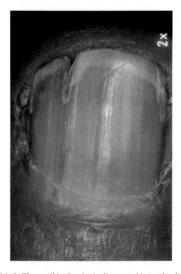

Figure 11.4 The nail in Darier's disease. Note the longitudinal bands and V-shaped notching.

Tuberous sclerosis complex

Tuberous sclerosis complex (TSC) is the preferred name for what was previously known as tuberous sclerosis or epiloia (*epi*lepsy, *lo*w *i*ntelligence and *a*denoma sebaceum). It is a dominantly inherited disorder, but many cases are sporadic and represent new mutations. In about half the cases the genetic abnormality occurs on chromosome 9q34 (TSC1) and in the others it is on chromosome 16p13 (TSC2).

There are hamartomatous malformations in the skin and internal organs. Characteristic skin lesions include numerous pink papules on the face (Fig. 11.5) (originally misleadingly called adenoma sebaceum), which are hamartomas of connective tissue and small blood vessels (angiofibromas); the 'shagreen' (having a resemblance to shark skin) patch on the back (a connective tissue naevus); periungual fibromas (Fig. 11.6); and hypopigmented macules (ash leaf macules) which are best seen with the aid of Wood's light. The hypopigmented macules are often present at birth, but the facial lesions usually first appear at the age of 5 or 6. Affected individuals may be mentally retarded and suffer from epilepsy. Other features include retinal phakomas, pulmonary and renal hamartomas, and cardiac rhabdomyomas.

Neurofibromatosis

There are two main forms of neurofibromatosis—type 1 (NF-1) (von Recklinghausen's disease) and type 2 (NF-2), both of which are of autosomal dominant inheritance. The gene for the more common type (NF-1) is located on chromosome 17q11.2 and that for NF-2 on chromosome 22q11.21. Both normally function as tumour suppressor genes.

NF-1 is characterized by multiple café-au-lait patches, axillary freckling (Crowe's sign), numerous neurofibromas (Fig. 11.7) and Lisch nodules (pigmented iris hamartomas). Other associated abnormalities include scoliosis, an increased risk of developing intracranial neoplasms, particularly optic nerve glioma, and an increased risk of hypertension associated with phaeochromocytoma or fibromuscular hyperplasia of the renal arteries.

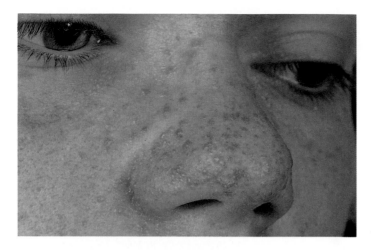

Figure 11.5 Facial angiofibromas in tuberous sclerosis.

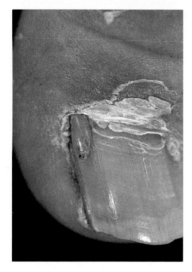

Figure 11.6 Periungual fibroma in tuberous sclerosis.

NF-2 is characterized by bilateral vestibular schwannomas (acoustic neuromas), as well as other central nervous system tumours.

Peutz–Jeghers syndrome

In this rare, dominantly inherited syndrome associated with mutations in a gene mapped to chromosome 19p13.3 there are pigmented macules (lentigines) in the mouth, on the lips, and on the hands and feet, in association with multiple hamartomatous intestinal polyps with low potential for malignant transformation.

Hereditary haemorrhagic telangiectasia (Osler–Weber–Rendu disease)

Mutations in at least two genes are responsible for this rare, dominantly inherited disorder in which numerous telangiectases are present on the face and lips and the nasal, buccal and intestinal mucosae. Recurrent epistaxes are common, and there is also a risk of gastointestinal haemorrhage. There is an association with pulmonary and cerebral arteriovenous fistulae. Visible vascular lesions can be treated with a laser.

Basal cell naevus syndrome (Gorlin's syndrome)

Gorlin's syndrome is an autosomal dominant disorder associated with mutations of the tumour-suppressor gene *PTCH* on chromosome 9q22.3–3.1. Multiple basal cell carcinomas (BCCs) on the face and trunk are associated with characteristic palmar pits, odontogenic keratocysts of the jaw, calcification of the falx cerebri, skeletal abnormalities and medulloblastoma.

The BCCs should be dealt with when they are small. Radiotherapy is contraindicated as this pro-

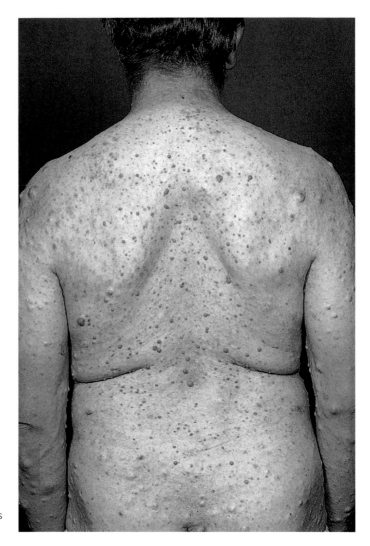

Figure 11.7 Von Recklinghausen's neurofibromatosis.

motes subsequent development of multiple lesions in the radiotherapy field.

Gardner's syndrome

This condition is also dominantly inherited. The gene responsible is located on chromosome 5q21–22, and it is thought that Gardner's syndrome and familial polyposis coli are allelic disorders caused by mutation in the *APC* (adenomatous polyposis coli) gene, which is another tumour-suppressor gene. Affected individuals have multiple epidermoid cysts, osteomas, and large-bowel adenomatous polyps that have a high risk of malignant change.

Ectodermal dysplasias

These are disorders in which there are defects of hair, teeth, nails or sweat glands. Most are extremely rare. One of the more common syndromes is hypohidrotic ectodermal dysplasia in which eccrine sweat glands are absent or markedly reduced in number; the scalp hair, eyebrows and eyelashes

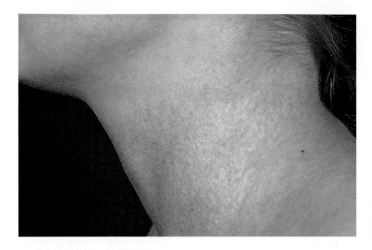

Figure 11.8 'Plucked chicken' appearance of the skin in pseudoxanthoma elasticum.

are sparse and the teeth are widely spaced and conical. The absence of sweating causes heat intolerance. It is inherited as an X-linked recessive trait.

Pseudoxanthoma elasticum (PXE)

Most cases of this disorder of connective tissue are recessively inherited. Results of recent work suggest that PXE is a primary metabolic disorder in which *MRP6/ABCC6* gene mutations lead to metabolic abnormalities that result in progressive calcification of elastic fibres. This affects elastic tissue in the dermis, blood vessels and Bruch's membrane in the eye. The skin of the neck and axillae has a lax 'plucked chicken' appearance of tiny yellowish papules (Fig. 11.8). Retinal angioid streaks, caused by ruptures in Bruch's membrane, are visible on fundoscopy. The abnormal elastic tissue in blood vessels may lead to gastrointestinal haemorrhage.

Xeroderma pigmentosum

Ultraviolet (UV) damage to epidermal DNA is normally repaired by an enzyme system. In xeroderma pigmentosum, which is recessively inherited, this system is defective, and UV damage is not repaired. This leads to the early development of skin cancers. Basal cell carcinomas, squamous cell carcinomas and malignant melanomas may all develop in childhood. In some cases, there is also gradual neurological deterioration caused by progressive neuronal loss.

Acrodermatitis enteropathica

In this recessively inherited disorder there is defective absorption of zinc. The condition is usually manifest in early infancy as exudative eczematous lesions around the orifices, and on the hands and feet. Affected infants also suffer from diarrhoea. Acrodermatitis enteropathica can be effectively treated with oral zinc supplements.

Angiokeratoma corporis diffusum (Anderson–Fabry disease)

This condition is the result of an inborn error of glycosphingolipid metabolism. It is inherited in an X-linked recessive manner. Deficiency of the enzyme alpha-galactosidase A leads to deposition of ceramide trihexoside in a number of tissues, including the cardiovascular system, the kidneys, the eyes and peripheral nerves. The skin lesions are tiny vascular angiokeratomas that are usually scattered over the lower trunk, buttocks, genitalia and thighs. Associated features caused by tissue deposition of the lipid include the following.

Anderson–Fabry disease

- Premature ischaemic heart disease
- Renal failure
- Severe pain and paraesthesiae in the hands and feet
- Corneal and lens opacities

Incontinentia pigmenti

An X-linked dominant disorder, incontinentia pigmenti occurs predominantly in female infants, as it is usually lethal *in utero* in males. Linear bullous lesions are present on the trunk and limbs at birth, or soon thereafter. The bullae are gradually replaced by warty lesions, and these in turn are eventually replaced by streaks and whorls of hyperpigmentation. Incontinentia pigmenti is frequently associated with a variety of ocular, skeletal, dental and central nervous system abnormalities.

Chromosomal abnormalities

Some syndromes caused by chromosomal abnormalities may have associated dermatological problems.

Associated dermatological problems

- Down's syndrome: increased incidence of alopecia areata and crusted scabies
- Turner's syndrome: primary lymphoedema
- Klinefelter's syndrome: premature venous ulceration
- XYY syndrome: premature venous ulceration; prone to develop severe nodulocystic acne

Chapter 12

Pigmentary disorders

Bold was her face, and fair, and red of hew.
(Chaucer, *The Wife of Bath*)

The complexion of the skin and the colour of the hair correspond to the colour of the moisture which the flesh attracts—white, or red, or black.
(Hippocrates)

Introduction: normal pigmentary mechanisms

Our skin colour is important, and there are many references to it in prose and poetry. We all note skin colour in our initial assessment of someone, and cutaneous pigment has been used to justify all manner of injustices. Any departure from the perceived norm can have serious psychological effects and practical implications.

A number of factors give rise to our skin colour.

Skin colour factors

- Haemoglobin
- Exogenous pigments in or on the skin surface
- Endogenously produced pigments (e.g. bilirubin)
- The pigments produced in the skin itself: melanin and phaeomelanin

The last two are the most important in dictating our basic skin colour

---

Normal pigmentary mechanisms have already been outlined in Chapter 1. Humans actually have a rather dull range of natural colours when com-

pared with peacocks, humming birds or parrots: normally only shades of brown and red. 'Brownness' is due to *melanin*, the intensity varying from almost white (no melanin) to virtually jet-black (lots). The genetics of melanin pigmentation is autosomal dominant.

Red is a bonus: only some people can produce *phaeomelanin*. Red is much more common in some races (e.g. Celts) than in others (e.g. Chinese).

Most human skin pigment is within keratinocytes, having been manufactured in melanocytes and transferred in melanosomes. There are racial differences in production, distribution and degradation of melanosomes, but not in the number of melanocytes (see Chapter 1). There are, however, important genetic differences, reflected in the response to ultraviolet (UV) radiation, conventionally called 'skin types'.

Skin types

- Type I —always burns, never tans
- Type II —burns easily, tans poorly
- Type III —burns occasionally, tans easily
- Type IV —never burns, tans easily
- Type V —genetically brown (e.g. Indian) or Mongoloid
- Type VI —genetically black (Congoid or Negroid)

The first response to UV radiation is an increased distribution of melanosomes. This rapidly increases basal layer pigmentation—the 'sun tan'. If stimulation is quickly withdrawn, as typically happens after 2 weeks on the Costa del Sol, the tan fades rapidly and peels off with normal epidermal turnover. If exposure is more prolonged, melanin production is stepped up more permanently. Tanning represents the skin's efforts to offer protection from the harmful effects of UV radiation, such as premature ageing and cancers.

We shall now look at states in which these pigmentary mechanisms appear to be abnormal, leading to decreased (hypo-) or increased (hyper-) pigmentation.

Hypopigmentation

Among the most important causes of hypopigmentation are the following.

Hypopigmentation causes
Congenital
• Albinism
• Phenylketonuria
• Tuberous sclerosis complex
• Hypochromic naevi
Acquired
• Vitiligo
• Sutton's halo naevi
• Tuberculoid leprosy
• Pityriasis (tinea) versicolor
• Pityriasis alba
• Lichen sclerosus
• Drugs and chemicals:
occupational leukoderma
self-inflicted/iatrogenic
• Postinflammatory hypopigmentation

Congenital

Some individuals are born with generalized or localized defects in pigmentation.

Albinism and *phenylketonuria* are due to defects in melanin production. In albinos, the enzyme tyrosinase may be *absent* (tyrosinase-negative) leading to generalized white skin and hair, and red eyes (the iris is also depigmented). Vision is usually markedly impaired, with nystagmus.

In some albinism, the enzyme is *defective* (tyrosinase-positive). The clinical picture is not as severe, and colour gradually increases with age. However,

skin cancers are very common in both forms. Albinism also illustrates the social importance of colour: in some societies, albinos are rejected and despised, in others they are revered.

The biochemical defect in phenylketonuria results in reduced tyrosine, the precursor of melanin, and increased phenylalanine (which inhibits tyrosinase). There is a generalized reduction of skin, hair and eye colour.

One of the cardinal signs of *tuberous sclerosis complex* (*epiloia*) is hypopigmented macules. These are often lanceolate (ash-leaf shaped), but may assume bizarre shapes. They are often the first signs of the disease. Any infant who presents with fits should be examined under Wood's light, as the macules can be seen more easily—see Chapter 2. Identical localized pale areas may occur without any other abnormality, when they are termed *hypochromic naevi*.

Acquired

Acquired hypopigmentation is common and, in darker skin, may have a particular stigma. This is partly because the cosmetic appearance of patchy hypopigmentation is much worse, but also because white patches are inextricably linked in some cultures with leprosy. Historically all white patches were probably classified as leprosy: Naaman (who was cured of 'leprosy' after bathing in the Jordan (2 Kings 5:1–14)) probably had vitiligo (see below).

Vitiligo is the most important cause of patches of pale skin. The skin in vitiligo becomes *de*pigmented and not hypopigmented, although during progression this is not always complete.

Characteristically there is complete loss of pigment from otherwise entirely normal skin (Fig. 12.1). Patches may be small, but commonly become large, often with irregular outlines. Depigmentation may spread to involve wide areas of the body. Although vitiligo can occur anywhere, it is often strikingly symmetrical, involving the hands, perioral and periocular skin.

The pathophysiology is poorly understood. In early patches, melanocytes are still present, but produce no melanin. Later, melanocytes disappear completely, except deep around hair follicles.

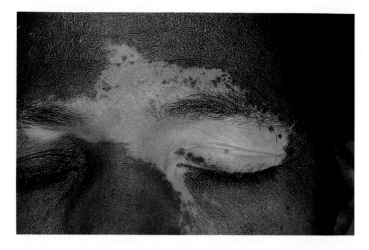

Figure 12.1 A typical patch of vitiligo.

Vitiligo may be an autoimmune process: there is an increase in organ-specific autoantibodies (as in alopecia areata, with which vitiligo may coexist).

Treatment is generally unsatisfactory. Topical steroids have their advocates, and PUVA can be successful. Some have claimed success with vitamin D analogues. Cosmetic camouflage may be helpful. Sun-screens should be used in the summer, because vitiliginous areas will not tan.

In some patients, particularly children, areas may repigment spontaneously. This is less common in adults and in longstanding areas. Repigmentation often begins with small dots coinciding with hair follicles. A similar appearance occurs in *Sutton's halo naevus* (see Chapter 10).

Some of the stigma associated with hypopigmentation is because *tuberculoid leprosy* is another cause. The (usually solitary) patch of hypopigmented skin also exhibits diminished sensation. Pale patches are also seen in the earliest stages: so-called 'indeterminate' leprosy.

The organism causing *pityriasis versicolor* (see Chapter 4) secretes azelaic acid. This results in hypopigmentation, most noticeably after sun exposure.

Pityriasis alba (a low-grade eczema) is a very common cause of hypopigmentation in children, especially in darker skins. Pale patches with a slightly scaly surface appear on the face and upper arms (Fig. 12.2). The condition usually responds (albeit slowly) to moisturizers, but may require mild topi-

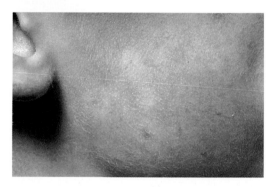

Figure 12.2 Pityriasis alba on the cheek.

cal steroids. The tendency appears to clear at puberty.

Lichen sclerosus (*et atrophicus*) (see Chapter 15) usually affects the genitalia. On other sites it is sometimes called 'white spot disease'.

Drugs and chemicals may cause loss of skin pigment. These may be encountered at work, but a more common source is skin lightening creams which, sadly, are all too commonly used by those with dark skin The active ingredient is generally hydroquinone, which can be used therapeutically (see below).

Many inflammatory skin disorders may produce secondary or *postinflammatory* hypopigmentation, due to a disturbance in the integrity of the epidermis and its melanin production: both eczema and psoriasis may leave temporary hypopigmentation when they resolve. However, inflammation can destroy melanocytes altogether: in scars, after burns and in areas treated with cryotherapy (it is the basis of 'freeze-branding').

Hyperpigmentation

As with hypopigmentation, there are many causes of increased skin pigmentation, including excessive production of melanin, or the deposition in the skin of several other pigments, such as beta-carotene, bilirubin, drugs and metals. The major causes are as follows:

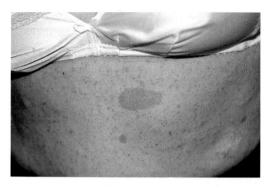

Figure 12.3 Café-au-lait patch in neurofibromatosis.

Causes of hyperpigmentation

Congenital
- Neurofibromatosis
- Peutz–Jeghers syndrome
- LEOPARD syndrome
- Incontinentia pigmenti

Acquired
- Urticaria pigmentosa
- Addison's disease
- Renal failure
- Haemochromatosis
- Liver disease
- Carotenaemia:
  idiopathic
  myxoedema
  pernicious anaemia
- Acanthosis nigricans
- Chloasma
- Drugs and chemicals
- Postinflammatory hyperpigmentation

Congenital

Hyperpigmentation is prominent in *neurofibromatosis*: café-au-lait marks (Fig. 12.3) and axillary freckling are common. Speckled lentiginous pigmentation is seen around the mouth and on the hands in the *Peutz–Jeghers syndrome*, and similar but more widespread lentigines may accompany a number of congenital defects in the *LEOPARD syndrome* (Lentigines, Electrocardiographic abnormalities, Ocular hypertelorism, Pulmonary stenosis, Abnormalities of the genitalia, Retardation of growth and Deafness.).

Incontinentia pigmenti is a rare congenital disorder which causes hyperpigmentation in a whorled pattern, preceded by blisters and hyperkeratotic lesions, and sometimes accompanied by other congenital abnormalities.

Acquired

Urticaria pigmentosa is most common in children, but may affect adults. There is a widespread eruption of indistinct brown marks which urticate if rubbed. The disorder is due to abnormal numbers of dermal mast cells.

Chloasma, or melasma, is much more common in women than men. A characteristic pattern of hyperpigmentation develops on the forehead, cheeks and chin (Fig. 12.4). Provoking factors include sunlight, pregnancy and the oral contraceptive pill, but chloasma may occur spontaneously. Treatment is difficult. Avoidance of precipitating factors (especially sunlight and oestrogens) may help. Topical hydroquinone preparations are sometimes used.

Various drugs and chemicals can cause cutaneous hyperpigmentation (see Chapter 21).

In *postinflammatory* hyperpigmentation, disruption of the lower layers of the epidermis results in deposition of melanin granules in the dermis (pigmentary incontinence). Many skin disorders do this, particularly in pigmented skin, but lichen planus is particularly troublesome. There is no useful treatment, but the pigmentation gradually fades with time.

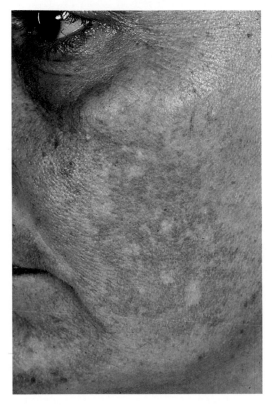

Figure 12.4 Typical chloasma.

Hyperpigmentation is an important physical sign in several systemic diseases:

1 *Addison's disease*—the changes are most marked in the skin creases, in scratch marks and in the gums.

2 *Renal failure*—may cause a muddy-brown skin colour.

3 *Haemochromatosis*—causes a deep golden-brown hue, diabetes and liver disease.

4 *Some chronic liver diseases*—result in deep pigmentation.

Beta-carotene (a yellow pigment) accumulates harmlessly in the skin in some normal individuals who ingest large amounts of carrots and orange juice (rich sources). The colour is most marked on the palms and soles. Similar deposition is seen in some patients with myxoedema and pernicious anaemia.

Another important, although rare, cause of acquired hyperpigmentation is *acanthosis nigricans*. This may or may not be associated with a systemic disease (see Chapter 19).

Chapter 13

Disorders of the hair and nails

If a woman have long hair, it is a glory to her. (St Paul (1 Corinthians, 11:15))

The hair takes root in the head at the same time as the nails grow. (Hippocrates)

Introduction

Hippocrates (see above) clearly knew that hair and nails were intimately connected, but there are many conditions which affect one or the other alone. We will deal with abnormalities of hair first and then nail disorders, but there will be some overlap.

Abnormalities of hair and nails may be the result of:

1 Local factors.
2 Generalized skin disease.
3 Systemic disease.

Hair abnormalities

Hair is important psychologically. Disturbances in growth or physical characteristics, even of minor degree, may be very upsetting: only Kojak really liked being bald! Remember that the distress caused is not necessarily proportionate to the severity apparent to an observer.

Patients present with three main hair abnormalities:

1 Changes in physical properties, such as colour or texture.

2 Thinning or loss of hair.
3 Excessive hair growth, including growth in abnormal sites.

Changes in physical properties of scalp hair

Common physical changes which are seen in hair are as follows:

Physical changes to hair

Pigmentation—greying/whiteness
• Genetic diseases, e.g. albinism, phenylketonuria
• Premature greying:
  physiological
  pathological, e.g. pernicious anaemia
• Ageing
• Vitiligo
• Alopecia areata

Textural abnormalities
• Brittleness
• Coarseness
• Curliness

Change in colour

Greying of the hair, whether premature or not, is permanent, including, usually, the white hair in scalp vitiligo. Regrowing hair in alopecia areata (see below) is often white initially, but often repigments later.

Textural abnormalities

Brittleness or coarseness may accompany hair thinning in hypothyroidism and in iron deficiency (see below). Hair may also become lack-lustre from hairdressing techniques (back-combing, bleaching and drying). In men, hair may become curly in the early stages of androgenetic alopecia (see below).

Scalp hair loss

Congenital disorders

Abnormal scalp hair loss is a feature of some congenital disorders.

Congenital disorders and scalp hair loss

- Ectodermal dysplasias
- Premature ageing syndromes
- Monilethrix
- Pili torti
- Marie–Unna alopecia
- Disorders of amino acid metabolism
- Scalp naevi (especially epithelial or organoid)
- Aplasia cutis

Very few of these conditions are amenable to treatment, but they require careful assessment, often including microscopic examination of hair shafts.

Acquired disorders

Patients most commonly seek advice about hair loss when it is from the scalp, although other areas may be affected. The most effective approach to the diagnosis of acquired scalp hair loss is:

1 to consider whether the changes are diffuse or circumscribed, and
2 to assess the state of the scalp skin.

When this information is combined with some knowledge of the disorders mentioned below, a preliminary diagnostic assessment can be made.

Telogen effluvium is often triggered by major illness, operations, accidents or other stress. A large percentage of hairs suddenly stop growing, enter the resting or 'telogen' phase, and start to fall out about 3 months later. Therefore, ask about any major upset in the appropriate period. Pull gently on hairs on the crown or sides, and several will come out easily: with a hand lens, the bulb looks much smaller than normal. Telogen effluvium should settle spontaneously, but can unmask androgenetic alopecia (see below), and some patients find their hair never returns completely to normal.

Appropriate tests will exclude important systemic diseases as a cause, and correct treatment may restore hair growth.

Acquired causes of scalp hair loss

Diffuse hair loss with normal scalp skin
- Telogen effluvium
- Thyroid disease
- Iron deficiency
- Drugs
- Systemic lupus erythematosus
- Secondary syphilis
- Alopecia totalis

Androgenetic alopecia
Circumscribed hair loss with normal scalp skin
- Alopecia areata
- Traction
- Trichotillomania

Hair loss with abnormal scalp skin
Without scarring
- Severe psoriasis or seborrhoeic dermatitis
- Tinea capitis (see Chapter 4)

With scarring
- Discoid lupus erythematosus
- Lichen planus
- Pseudopelade
- Cicatricial pemphigoid
- Lupus vulgaris

Many drugs can induce hair loss.

Drugs inducing hair loss

- Cytotoxic agents
- Antithyroid agents, especially thiouracil
- Anticoagulants
- Retinoids
- Thallium

All of these processes can be confused with alopecia areata (see below) when the latter is widespread and rapidly progressive.

Androgenetic alopecia (or common balding) occurs in both men and women. It is due to the effects of androgens in genetically susceptible individuals.

In men, the process may begin at any age after puberty; however, it is much more common from the thirties onwards and, by age 70, 80% show some hair loss. Hair is usually lost first at the temples and/or on the crown, but there may be complete hair loss, sparing a rim at the back and sides. Terminal hairs become progressively finer and smaller, until only a few vellus hairs remain. The extent and pace vary widely.

In women, the process is slower and less severe, but causes much distress. Up to half of all women have mild hair loss on the vertex by age 50, and, in some, more severe thinning occurs. There may be accompanying hirsutism (see below).

Until recently there was no known treatment, but there is some evidence that early use of topical minoxidil may help both men and women, and relatively selective antiandrogenic agents (e.g. finasteride) are becoming available.

Circumscribed hair loss with normal scalp skin

Alopecia areata

The cause of this disorder is unknown but it is probably an autoimmune process. As in vitiligo (see Chapter 12), organ-specific autoantibodies (to thyroid, adrenal or gastric parietal cells) are often found in the patients' sera.

History. One or more areas of baldness suddenly appear on the scalp, in the eyebrows, beard or elsewhere. It is most common in childhood and early adult life, although periodic recurrences may happen at any age.

Examination. Patches are typically round or oval (Fig. 13.1); the skin usually appears completely normal, although there may be mild erythema; a number of areas may develop next to each other, giving rise to a moth-eaten appearance; close examination of the edge of a patch of alopecia areata reveals the pathognomonic feature—'exclamation mark hairs'—short hairs which taper towards the base (Fig. 13.2).

Prognosis. Most patches regrow after a few weeks, although further episodes are common; initial hair growth may be white; occasionally, the process spreads and may become permanent—if this state

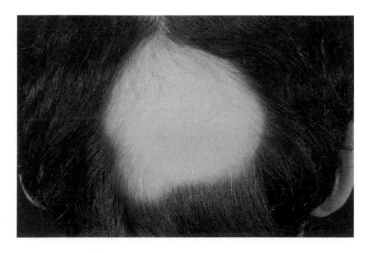

Figure 13.1 A typical patch of alopecia areata.

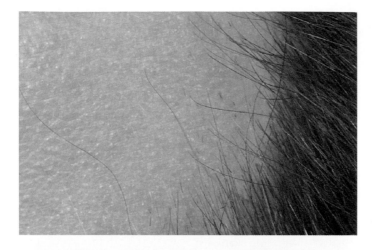

Figure 13.2 The edge of the area seen in Figure 13.1. Exclamation mark hairs are visible at the margin.

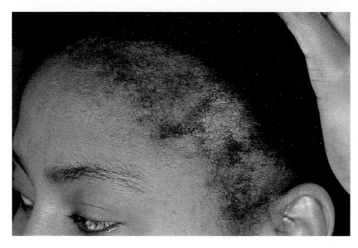

Figure 13.3 Traction alopecia.

involves the whole scalp it is termed *alopecia totalis* and if the whole body is affected, the name *alopecia universalis* is applied. The nails may be affected in severe cases (see below).

Treatment. This is difficult, but intralesional steroids may help, and topical sensitizers such as diphencyprone are also used.

Chronic traction can also cause circumscribed alopecia, often around scalp margins (Fig. 13.3). It is commonly seen in young girls with tight pony tails, Sikh boys, and Afro-Caribbean children whose hair is dressed in multiple little pigtails.

In *trichotillomania*, hair is pulled, twisted or rubbed out, and affected site(s) are covered in broken hairs of different lengths. There may be psychological factors (see Chapter 20).

Hair loss with abnormal scalp skin

Psoriasis, seborrhoeic dermatitis and other inflammatory processes can cause temporary hair loss: an important cause is tinea capitis (see Chapter 4).

In some conditions, fibrosis accompanies the inflammation, and this may result in permanent damage to hair follicles, and obvious loss of tissue or atrophy. This is known as *scarring* or *cicatricial* alopecia.

Examination of the rest of the skin may provide important clues.

Causes of cicatricial alopecia

Discoid lupus erythematosus
- Prominent plugging of the hair follicles
- Look for lesions on the face

Lichen planus
- May accompany lichen planus elsewhere
- Nail involvement is common (see Chapter 15)

Cicatricial pemphigoid
- Alopecia follows blistering

Lupus vulgaris (cutaneous TB)
- Especially in international residents

Trigeminal trophic syndrome
- May follow herpes zoster because of hypoaesthesia and chronic trauma

Pseudopelade
- Small patches of scarring alopecia without distinguishing features

In most of these conditions, a biopsy is essential. In cases where lupus erythematosus or cicatricial pemphigoid are suspected, immunofluorescence should also be performed.

Generalized hair loss

Generalized hair loss is rare, but may accompany endocrine disturbances, especially *hypothyroidism* or *hypopituitarism*. Drugs, particularly cytotoxics, may induce widespread alopecia. As has been mentioned, alopecia areata may lead to complete hair loss—*alopecia universalis*.

Excessive hair and hair in abnormal sites

Hirsutism

This term is applied to excessive growth of hair in a female, distributed in a male secondary sexual pattern.

A search for more serious causes is indicated if the changes are of rapid onset.

Causes of hirsutism

- Mild hirsutism is quite common in elderly women
- It may be a genetic trait in younger females, when the changes may accompany a general reduction in scalp hair (see androgenetic alopecia above)
- Minor endocrine disturbances, especially polycystic ovary syndrome
- Drugs with androgenic activity
- Virilizing tumours

Treatment includes shaving, waxing, depilatory creams, electrolysis and laser ablation. The antiandrogen cyproterone acetate may help.

Hypertrichosis

Excessive hair growth in a non-sexual distribution may occur in both sexes. There are several causes:

Causes of hypertrichosis

- Congenital generalized, e.g. Cornelia de Lange syndrome
- Congenital localized, e.g. 'faun-tail' in spina bifida occulta
- Drugs such as:
  minoxidil (now used for baldness—see above)
  ciclosporin (cyclosporin)
  hydantoins
  systemic steroids
- Anorexia nervosa
- Cachexia
- Porphyria cutanea tarda: associated with scarring and milia
- Pretibial myxoedema: overlying plaques

Nail abnormalities

Nail changes may be non-specific, or characteristic of specific processes. They may occur in isolation, but the nails are abnormal in several disorders.

Disorders with abnormal nails

Congenital
- Especially disorders of keratinization, e.g. Darier's disease
- Ectodermal dysplasias
- Due to scarring, e.g. dystrophic epidermolysis bullosa

Acquired
- Psoriasis
- Eczema/dermatitis
- Lichen planus
- Alopecia areata/totalis
- Fungal infections

Common nail abnormalities

Brittleness
- Increases with age
- Seen in iron deficiency (see also koilonychia) and thyroid disease

Roughness (trachyonychia)
- Common and often non-specific
- May result from widespread pitting (see below)

Beau's lines
- Horizontal grooves which follow a major illness

Pits
- Classical feature of psoriasis
- Severe alopecia areata (smaller, more evenly distributed than in psoriasis)
- Eczema/dermatitis (coarse dents and irregular pits)

Onycholysis
- Lifting of nail plate off nail bed
- Causes:
  psoriasis
  fungal infection (see Chapter 4)
  thyrotoxicosis
  space-occupying lesion (e.g. exostosis or tumour)
- May be no other identifiable abnormality present

Clubbing
- Sign of pulmonary, liver or thyroid disease; may be familial

Discoloration
- White marks—common normal variant
- White nails—associated with cirrhosis
- Pale—anaemia
- Half red/half pale—renal disease
- Sulfur yellow—fungal infection
- Uniform yellow—'yellow nail syndrome' (+bronchiectasis and lymphoedema)
- Green-blue—*Pseudomonas* infection
- Brown-black—melanoma, haematoma
- Linear brown—naevus

Koilonychia
- Nails with a concave upper surface (spoon-shaped)
- Causes:
  iron deficiency
  inherited

Washboard nails (Fig. 13.4)
- Habitual picking of nail fold leads to surface ridging

Onychogryphosis
- Grossly thickened, distorted nails (Fig. 13.5) often due to neglect

'Pterygium'
- Damage leads to epithelium encroaching on nail surface
- Most common cause—lichen planus

Loss of nails
- Causes:
  pterygium
  scarring, e.g. Stevens–Johnson syndrome
  severe inflammation, e.g. pustular psoriasis

Common disorders of the paronychium

Patients may also complain of disorders of the area around the nail—the paronychium.

Paronychia

There are two common forms, acute and chronic. In acute paronychia, an abscess in the nail fold forms, points and discharges. It is nearly always staphylococcal. Chronic paronychia is discussed in Chapter 4.

Ingrowing nails

Overcurved nails (especially on big toes) dig into the lateral nail fold leading to chronic inflammation and overproduction of granulation tissue. Sometimes this can be prevented by trimming nails straight, but surgical intervention is often required.

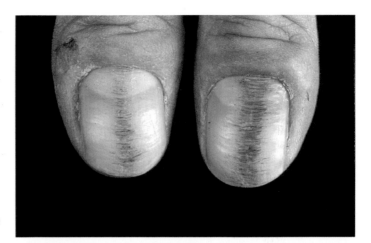

Figure 13.4 'Washboard' nails on the thumbs: the result of a habit tic.

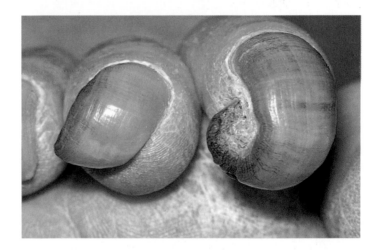

Figure 13.5 Onychogryphosis.

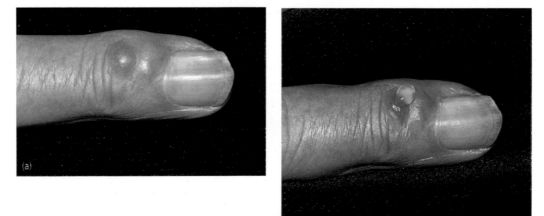

Figure 13.6 (a) Myxoid cyst of the finger. (b) Insertion of a needle releases crystal-clear, gelatinous contents.

Periungual warts

Warts are discussed in Chapter 3. Periungual warts are unsightly and extremely difficult to eradicate.

Myxoid cyst

Small cystic swellings may appear on the proximal nail fold (Fig. 13.6). The nail may develop a linear depression. Clear gelatinous fluid can be expressed, if the surface is breached (Fig 13.6b). These cysts are more common in middle-aged and elderly people. A myxoid cyst is essentially a ganglion connected to the distal interphalangeal joint by a narrow pedicle. Treatment is with cryotherapy, or various surgical procedures.

Chapter 14

Bullous disorders

All that blisters is not pemphigus (Graham-Brown and Burns, 1990)

Causes

The skin has a limited repertoire of changes, but few are more dramatic than an eruption of blisters or bullae. There are many causes.

This is a fairly comprehensive differential diagnostic list for further reading. Some disorders, such as impetigo and the viral causes, are mentioned elsewhere. This chapter deals with the most important remaining causes of blistering.

Causes of bullae

Physical injury
- Cold, heat, friction
- Severe oedema

Infections (see Chapters 3 and 4)
Bacterial
- Impetigo

Viral
- Chickenpox
- Herpes zoster
- Herpes simplex
- Smallpox and vaccinia
- Hand, foot and mouth disease

Fungal
- Tinea pedis with pompholyx

Arthropods (see Chapter 5)
- Insect bites

Drugs (see also Chapter 21)
- Barbiturates, sulfonamides, iodides, frusemide (furosemide), nalidixic acid (light-induced)
- Drug-induced pemphigus and pemphigoid
- Fixed drug eruptions

Skin disorders
Congenital
- Epidermolysis bullosa

Acquired
Bullae are a major feature in:
- Pemphigus
- Bullous pemphigoid
- Cicatricial pemphigoid
- Dermatitis herpetiformis
- Linear IgA disease
- Epidermolysis bullosa acquisita
- Toxic epidermal necrolysis
Bullae may occur in:
- Erythema multiforme (Stevens–Johnson syndrome)
- Eczema (including pompholyx)
- Lichen planus
- Psoriasis (pustular)
- Vasculitis

Metabolic disease
- Porphyria cutanea tarda, diabetes mellitus

Physical causes of bullae

Burns may result from cold, heat or chemical injury and are a common cause of blisters, as is extreme friction (e.g. the feet of vigorous squash players or joggers).

Oedema

Severe oedema of the lower legs may also produce tense bullae.

Arthropods

Remember that insect bites very commonly present as tense bullae (see Chapter 5). In the UK, this is most common in late summer and early autumn (fall).

Drugs

Several drugs cause blistering (see above). Blisters caused by nalidixic acid occur on the lower legs following sun exposure. Fixed drug eruptions may blister (see Chapter 21).

Skin disorders

Primary skin disorders giving rise to bullae may be congenital or acquired. In some, bullae are an important or integral part of the clinical presentation. In others, blisters may occur but are not the most prominent or constant feature, and the reader should consult the appropriate chapter for further information.

Congenital

Epidermolysis bullosa

Although very rare, this is an important group of disorders. Babies are born with fragile skin that blisters on contact. There are several variants, with splits at different levels in the skin; all are unpleasant and some are fatal.

Diagnosis requires electron microscopy to determine the level of the blister.

The differential diagnosis of blistering in a neonate must also include a number of other disorders:
1 Impetigo (pemphigus neonatorum).
2 Staphylococcal scalded skin syndrome (see below).
3 Incontinentia pigmenti (see Chapter 11).

Acquired

Pemphigus

The cardinal pathological processes in all forms of pemphigus are:
1 A split within the epidermis.
2 Loss of adhesion of epidermal cells ('acantholysis').

These changes may be just above the basal layer (pemphigus vulgaris; Fig. 14.1) or higher in the epidermis (pemphigus foliaceus; Fig. 14.2).

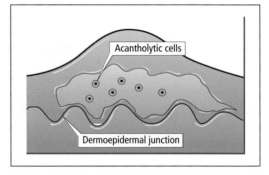

Figure 14.1 Pemphigus vulgaris: split just above the basal layer, with overlying acantholysis of epidermal cells.

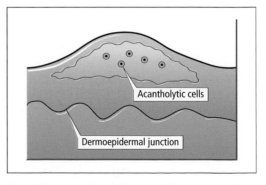

Figure 14.2 Pemphigus foliaceus: similar changes to those in Figure 14.1 but higher in the epidermis.

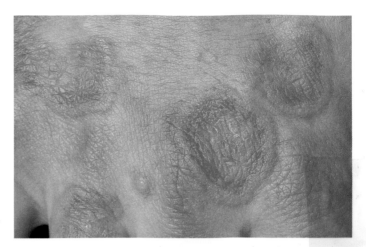

Figure 15.3 'Target' lesions of erythema multiforme.

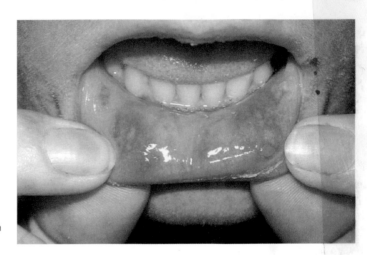

Figure 15.4 Erosions on the lips in bullous erythema multiforme.

Exfoliative dermatitis (erythroderma)

These terms (either will do) are used to describe a state in which most of the skin becomes red, inflamed and scaly (Fig. 15.5).

The correct management depends on the underlying disease process, because the optimum treatment is different. The four most important causes of exfoliative dermatitis are:

- Psoriasis.
- Eczema/dermatitis.
- Drug reactions.
- Lymphomas (especially cutaneous T-cell lymphoma).

Clinical features. The skin is red, hot and scaly; there may be generalized lymphadenopathy; there is a loss of control of temperature regulation, and there are bouts of shivering as the body attempts to compensate for heat loss by generating metabolic heat.

Effects. Cardiac output is increased; protein is lost from the skin (and the gut); water loss from the skin is increased; patients radiate heat into their surroundings; there is a rise in metabolic rate, with mobilization of energy sources and increased muscle activity; the body cannot compensate for long, especially in elderly patients.

135

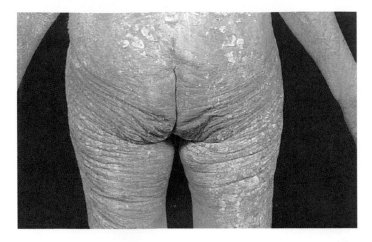

Figure 15.5 Exfoliative dermatitis.

Complications. Cardiac failure; renal failure; sudden death due to central hypothermia.

Treatment
1 Stop any potential causative drugs (see Chapter 21).
2 Nurse the patient in a warm room.
3 Attend to secondary medical problems (e.g. dehydration, heart failure and infections).
4 Biopsy skin to obtain definitive diagnosis.
5 Give a short course of systemic steroids (if the diagnosis is known to be psoriasis from the outset, commence systemic antipsoriatic drugs instead— see Chapter 8).
6 Initiate appropriate treatment for underlying diagnosis.

Lichen planus

Lichen planus is a rather variable disorder, said to affect 1% of new referrals to a dermatologist. The most common pattern is an acute eruption of itchy papules (Fig. 15.6).

Sites of predilection. Wrists, ankles and the small of the back, mouth and genitalia.

Clinical features
1 Skin lesions:
   (a) flat-topped;
   (b) shiny;
   (c) polygonal (Fig. 15.6).

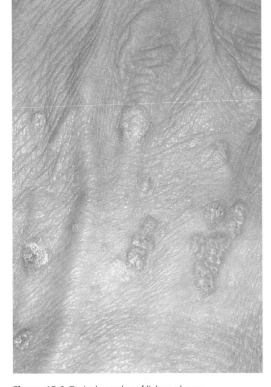

Figure 15.6 Typical papules of lichen planus.

2 Surface—fine network of dots or lines called 'Wickham's striae'.
3 Colour—'violaceous' (reddish-purple).
4 Oral—lacy, reticulate streaks on the cheeks (Fig. 15.7), gums and lips.

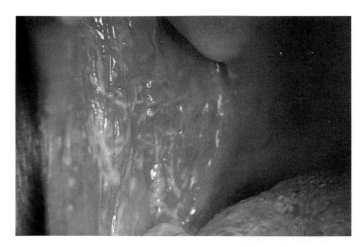

Figure 15.7 Oral lesions in lichen planus.

In the majority of patients, the eruption settles over a period of a few months. There are a number of variants, some of which are more persistent.

Aetiology. Lichen planus is a T-cell-mediated attack on the epidermis, similar changes being seen in graft-versus-host reactions. However, the cause of lichen planus in most instances remains a mystery.

Variants of lichen planus

- Hypertrophic: lichenified lumps appear on the legs
- Atrophic: largely seen in the mouth, lesions may be very chronic; small risk of carcinoma
- Follicular: may result in permanent scarring and hair loss
- Nail disease: nail changes may be very slight, or may lead to complete nail loss
- Drug-induced: see Chapter 21

Treatment. Potent topical steroids usually suppress irritation; very extensive or severe oral disease may need systemic steroids or ciclosporin.

Lichen nitidus

Probably a variant of lichen planus, this uncommon disorder produces clusters of tiny, asymptomatic papules.

Lichen sclerosus (et atrophicus)

Lichen sclerosus (previously called lichen sclerosus et atrophicus) is a disorder of unknown aetiology. *Sites of predilection.* The genitalia, especially in women.

Clinical features
1 White, atrophic patches on the vulva, perineum and perianal skin (Fig 15.8), or glans penis and foreskin.
2 Similar plaques may develop elsewhere.
3 Purpura and blistering may appear.
4 Vulval lichen sclerosus easily becomes eroded and haemorrhagic, with severe soreness and irritation.

Complications. Vulvo-vaginal stenosis; development of squamous cell carcinoma.

Childhood disease. Lichen sclerosus in prepubertal girls often presents with dysuria and pain on defaecation. It may be misdiagnosed as sexual abuse, but lesions are usually easy to diagnose, and parents and child can be reassured. The prognosis of childhood disease is good, as many clear at puberty.

Disease in males. Lichen sclerosus may be seen on the glans and prepuce (sometimes called 'balanitis xerotica obliterans'), and can give rise to phimosis

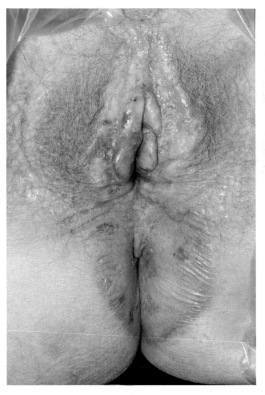

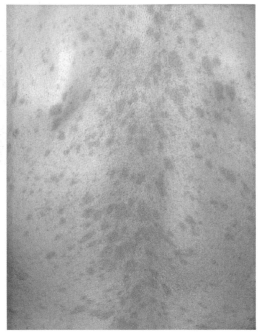

Figure 15.9 Pityriasis rosea.

Figure 15.8 Characteristic appearance of vulval lichen sclerosus.

and meatal stenosis. A significant number of boys undergo circumcision because of phimosis due to lichen sclerosus. There is a risk of squamous cell carcinoma. Extragenital lesions may also occur.

Treatment. The disease in adults generally pursues a chronic, relapsing course. Very potent topical steroids provide symptomatic relief in vulval disease, and clobetasol propionate is the treatment of choice. Patients should be kept under surveillance because of the risk of neoplastic change.

Pityriasis rosea

Pityriasis rosea is a self-limiting disorder, predominantly affecting children and young adults.

Clinical features
1 There may be a mild prodromal illness.

2 One or more 'herald patches' appear. A herald patch is large, red, oval and scaly, and usually appears on the trunk or upper arm (often misdiagnosed, especially as ringworm!).
3 A few days later, there is a sudden eruption of pink, oval patches on the trunk, upper arms and thighs.
There are three especially notable features:
1 On the trunk, lesions largely lie with their long axes in lines sweeping from the back to the front (almost as if they were following spinal nerves). This is said to resemble an 'inverted Christmas tree' (Fig. 15.9)—but that depends on your concept of a Christmas tree! However, once understood, this sign will never be forgotten and *no other disorder produces this*.
2 The scale on the surface of each lesion peels from the centre towards the edge, resulting in a so-called 'peripheral collarette' (Fig. 15.10).
3 If the diagnosis has still not been made, it becomes clear when the rash disappears (as it always does) in 6–8 weeks.

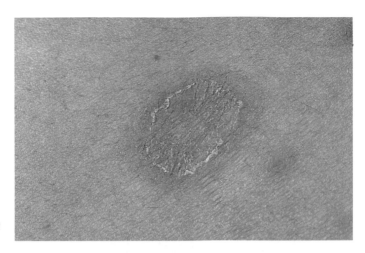

Figure 15.10 Pityriasis rosea: the 'peripheral collarette' of scale.

Treatment. Usually unnecessary, but mild topical steroids may help to relieve irritation.

Atypical pityriasis rosea

There may be no gap between the herald patch and the generalized rash; the eruption may extend down the arms and legs, and occasionally spares the trunk altogether; lesions may be so numerous that the distribution described above is not apparent; the inflammation may be so intense that it causes blisters.

Pityriasis lichenoides

Small brownish-red papules surmounted by a 'plate' of scale appear on the trunk and limbs. Some patients have more acutely inflamed lesions that heal to leave pock marks.

Pityriasis rubra pilaris

Pityriasis rubra pilaris (PRP) occurs in localized or generalized forms. All types are rare. Lesions are reddish-orange, and hair follicles are prominently involved. Generalized change is a very rare cause of exfoliative dermatitis (see above).

Miliaria or 'prickly heat'

This is the exotic name for little red bumps that some people develop in hot humid conditions. It is due to sweat duct obstruction. It should not be confused with polymorphic light eruption (see below), which is often erroneously called prickly heat, but in which the lesions are induced by light *not* heat. The condition is also seen in infants, particularly in the napkin area.

Pregnancy rashes

Pregnancy may alter the course of a number of skin disorders, such as acne, eczema, psoriasis and vulval warts, and it may trigger erythema multiforme.

There are also three important conditions related to pregnancy itself.

Conditions related to pregnancy

Pruritus of pregnancy
• Up to 20% of women; may be due to oestrogen-induced cholestasis

Polymorphic eruption of pregnancy
• Blotchy, urticarial and papular rash with intense itching
• Onset in third trimester
• Lesions favour abdomen
• Particular predilection for striae (Fig. 15.11)
• Fades shortly after delivery

Herpes (pemphigoid) gestationis
• Blisters on urticated background
• Variant of bullous pemphigoid
• Rare

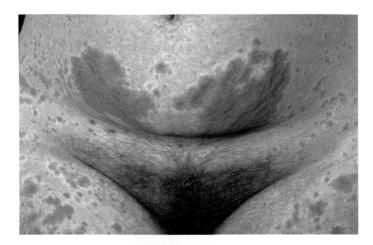

Figure 15.11 Polymorphic eruption of pregnancy.

Light-induced skin disease

But yet the light that led astray
Was light from Heaven
(Robert Burns, *The Vision*)

Sunlight is generally thought to be beneficial: adverts for sunbeds, solaria and foreign holidays all bear witness to this twentieth-century myth. However, ultraviolet (UV) radiation can initiate, wholly or in part, many unwanted skin changes:

• Some are chronic: cancers and keratoses (see Chapter 9); the yellowing, coarsening and wrinkling known as 'photo-ageing'. Note that most of today's tanned beauties are tomorrow's wrinkled prunes!
• Some are more acute: sunburn; reactions to a combination of plants or drugs and light.
• Some are due to metabolic disturbances, whereas in others the cause is quite unknown.

UV radiation may also exacerbate certain pre-existing skin disorders (see below).

Sunburn

Most of us are familiar with sunburn, even if only in others. Excessive medium wavelength UV radiation induces erythema and, if severe, blistering. The dose required depends on skin type (see Chapter 12), and the intensity of the UV radiation: skin

types I and II are very prone to sunburn; sunlight around midday is the most intense.

Treatment of established sunburn is difficult, but calamine lotion and topical steroids may help symptomatically. Prevention is much better than cure.

Sun care should include avoidance of intense exposure, hats and clothing, sunglasses and sun-screens. Exposed surfaces should be covered as far as possible. Sun-screens come in a range of potencies, graded by sun protection factor (SPF) number. This number indicates the approximate multiple of time to redness that the agent will provide: if the exposure time to redness is normally 10 min, SPF 6 sun-screen will prolong this to about an hour.

Unwanted cutaneous reactions to light

• Sunburn
• Polymorphic light eruption
• Solar urticaria (see above)
• Actinic prurigo
• Juvenile spring eruption
• Hydroa vacciniforme
• Photosensitive eczema
• Porphyrias
• Pellagra
• Xeroderma pigmentosum
• Phytophotodermatitis
• Drug reactions

Polymorphic light eruption

Frequently misdiagnosed as 'prickly heat' (see above), this affects women more often than men, and typically trouble starts in adolescence or early adulthood.

Clinical features. An eruption develops on light-exposed surfaces, most commonly the face, arms, legs and the 'V' of the neck. Individual lesions vary from papules to plaques. Blisters are sometimes seen. The reaction may only occur in very strong sunlight, but even mild British summer sunshine can be the trigger.

Treatment. Preseason PUVA is helpful. Antimalarials may be of some benefit, and sun-screens and clothing will help prevent the eruption.

Actinic prurigo

Actinic prurigo is a rare disorder of childhood in which eczematous areas develop on the face and backs of the hands every summer, and disappear in the winter. The cause is unknown, and attempted treatment is often ineffective.

Juvenile spring eruption

Little boys occasionally develop blisters on the ears in spring, and this is given the grand title of 'juvenile spring eruption'. It is probably a variant of polymorphic light eruption.

Photosensitive eczema and chronic actinic dermatitis

Some individuals develop eczema of light-exposed surfaces. In others, a pre-existing eczema becomes much worse on exposure to light.

One cause is a contact dermatitis to airborne chemicals, such as perfumes or plant extracts (e.g. chrysanthemums). A similar picture may occur with drugs.

The changes tend to become more intense until the skin is permanently thickened and inflamed. This state is termed 'chronic actinic dermatitis'.

Treatment. This is very difficult. Barrier sun-screens containing titanium may help, and azathioprine has been shown to be of benefit.

Porphyrias

This miscellaneous group of disorders is due to enzyme defects in the haem production pathways. Some, but not all, are associated with photosensitivity.

The most common in northern Europe is erythropoietic protoporphyria, in which burning in the sun (even through glass) develops in early childhood. A form known as 'variegate porphyria' is seen in some Dutch and South African pedigrees.

It is perhaps worth mentioning that one of the rarest porphyrias (congenital erythropoietic porphyria or Günther's disease) may be the origin of the werewolf legend. Sufferers become disfigured, hairy and anaemic (hence the werewolf's craving for blood). They avoid sunlight because of severe photosensitivity (the werewolf prowls at night when the moon is full—a logical time to prowl if there is no other source of illumination!).

Pellagra

A photosensitive rash in the malnourished should suggest pellagra. In Western societies the classical triad of diarrhoea, dermatitis and dementia is only seen in alcoholics and recluses.

Xeroderma pigmentosum

This rare disorder often presents with photosensitivity in early childhood (see also Chapter 11).

Phytophotodermatitis

Every summer, we see patients who have developed a rash following contact with plants on sunny days. Linear, streaky dermatitis (Fig. 15.12) results, and residual pigmentary disturbances are common. One important cause is giant hogweed, but there are several others.

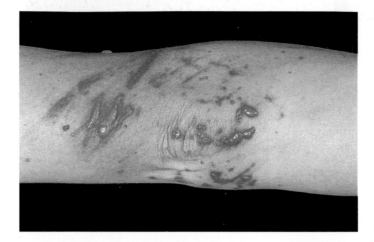

Figure 15.12 A phytophotodermatitis.

Light-induced drug reactions

Several groups of drugs are associated with photoallergic and phototoxic reactions (see Chapter 21).

Disorders exacerbated by light

A number of disorders may show a deterioration or provocation on exposure to light. The mechanisms for this are unclear.

Disorders exacerbated by light

- Lupus erythematosus
- Rosacea
- Psoriasis
- Darier's disease
- Herpes simplex

Chapter 16

Vascular disorders

Leg ulcers

By far the most common type of leg ulcer is the venous ulcer. Other causes of leg ulceration include ischaemia, vasculitis, skin neoplasia and certain haematological disorders.

Venous leg ulcers

Venous return from the legs is dependent on the deep and superficial venous systems and activity of the calf muscles. When the calf muscles contract, they pump blood in the deep veins towards the heart against gravity. Valves in the deep veins prevent reflux of blood when the muscles relax. During relaxation of the calf muscles, blood passes from the superficial veins into the deep veins via the sapheno-femoral and sapheno-popliteal junctions and numerous perforating veins. If the valves in the deep veins are incompetent, the calf muscle pump cannot function effectively and venous hypertension develops. Congenital abnormalities of the venous system, and valve damage following deep vein thrombosis, contribute to incompetence. Genetic factors are important as certain racial groups have a low prevalence of venous hypertension and venous ulcers.

The high pressure in the deep veins of the legs is transmitted via incompetent perforating veins to the superficial venous system (resulting in 'varicose' veins), and eventually to the capillary network. Skin capillaries become dilated and tortuous, and there is increased transudation of fluid into the surrounding tissues. Fibrinogen in the transudate is converted to fibrin, which forms cuffs around blood vessels. Transfer of oxygen and nutrients to the surrounding tissues is impeded, and the relatively ischaemic tissues are susceptible to ulceration, either spontaneously or following minor trauma. This 'fibrin cuff' theory is only one of the proposed mechanisms for tissue ischaemia in venous hypertension, and the pathomechanics of ulceration have not been fully elucidated.

Problems caused by venous hypertension usually present in middle or old age, and women, particularly if obese, are predominantly affected. The clinical features are as follows.

Venous hypertension: clinical features

- Varicose veins
- Oedema
- Lipodermatosclerosis
- Hyperpigmentation
- Eczema
- Atrophie blanche
- Ulceration

Lipodermatosclerosis. This term refers to areas of induration, caused by fibrosis, on the lower parts of the legs, above the ankles (Fig. 16.1). There is initially an area of erythema, and this subsequently becomes purple-brown in colour. On palpation,

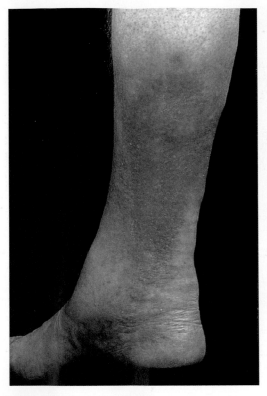

Figure 16.1 Lipodermatosclerosis.

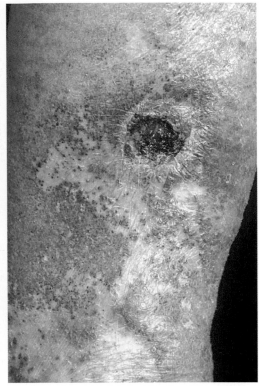

Figure 16.2 Atrophie blanche.

affected areas feel indurated. When the process is circumferential the tissues around the ankle are constricted and the leg above is oedematous, producing the classical 'inverted champagne bottle' appearance.

Hyperpigmentation. Haemosiderin, derived from red cells extravasated from dilated, leaky capillaries, produces areas of brown discoloration.

Eczema. Areas of 'varicose' eczema are common.

Atrophie blanche. This term is applied to areas of scar tissue within which are prominent dilated capillaries. Scattered pink dots are seen on a white background (Fig. 16.2). Such areas are very prone to ulcerate, and the ulcers are usually extremely painful.

Ulcers. The most common site for a venous ulcer is the medial aspect of the leg, just above the medial malleolus (Fig. 16.3), but the lateral malleolar area may also be affected.

Rarely, a squamous cell carcinoma may develop in a longstanding venous ulcer (Marjolin's ulcer).

Treatment

Varicose eczema may be treated with mild topical steroids. Colour Doppler duplex sonography should be performed, and assessment by a vascular surgeon is an important aspect of management, as some patients benefit significantly from surgery on incompetent superficial veins. In addition, it is essential to assess the arterial supply in patients with leg ulcers because they may have a remediable arterial abnormality. It is not uncommon to discover both venous and arterial pathology in individuals with leg ulcers.

Another essential component of the management of venous ulcers is reduction of venous hyper-

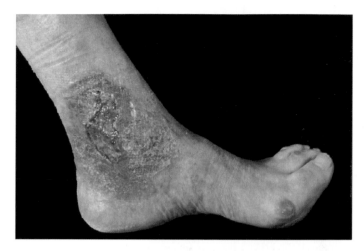

Figure 16.3 Venous ulcer.

tension and oedema by compression bandaging, which improves calf muscle pump function and opposes gravitational venous reflux. It is vital, however, to establish that the arterial supply to a limb is adequate (by assessing the ankle-brachial pressure index (ABPI) and by Doppler studies) before using compression bandaging.

Secondary infection, often with a mixed bacterial flora, occurs in the majority of venous ulcers. However, systemic antibiotic therapy is not necessary unless there is associated cellulitis (see Chapter 3).

There are numerous agents which have been marketed as topical therapies for leg ulcers, including alginate, hydrogel and hydrocolloid dressings, but a simple regimen of regular irrigation with saline and the application of a low-adherence dressing is adequate in many cases, if combined with compression bandaging. The most important concept to remember is that unless an effort is made to deal with the primary problem by compression bandaging and vein surgery when indicated, it doesn't matter what magical agent is applied to the ulcer because it won't heal.

When a venous ulcer has healed it is important to maintain compression by wearing appropriate compression hosiery.

Ischaemic ulcers

Ischaemic ulceration is usually a manifestation of atherosclerotic peripheral vascular disease. Typically, ischaemic ulcers occur on the dorsum or the sides of the foot, between the toes or on the heel, in an individual with a history of intermittent claudication and, later, rest pain. There are usually associated risk factors such as smoking, hypertension and diabetes. Pedal pulses are reduced or absent, and Doppler studies will demonstrate impaired blood flow. Ischaemic ulcers are usually painful.

The advice of a vascular surgeon should be sought.

Vasculitic ulcers

Vasculitis associated with a number of disorders, including rheumatoid arthritis and systemic lupus erythematosus (SLE), may produce leg ulcers.

Neoplastic ulcers

Basal cell carcinomas and squamous cell carcinomas arising on the legs may resemble, and be mistaken for, venous ulcers. However, they usually occur above the ankle region. If there is any suspicion that an ulcer is neoplastic, a biopsy should be performed.

Haematological disorders and leg ulcers

Uncommon causes of leg ulcers include hereditary spherocytosis, sickle cell anaemia and thalassaemia. The mechanism of ulceration in these conditions is related to tissue hypoxia due to blockage of skin capillaries by abnormally shaped red cells.

Vasculitis

Vasculitis is an inflammatory process affecting blood vessels. There have been several attempts at classification of vasculitis and none has proved entirely satisfactory, but systems employed are usually based on the size of vessel involved and the histological features. Recently proposed classifications have two major categories—small and larger vessel vasculitides. However, if you are tempted to explore vasculitis in depth and find the subject confusing, don't worry, so does everyone else.

Factors involved in the pathogenesis of vasculitis include immune complexes, in which the antigens are of bacterial, viral or drug origin, antineutrophil cytoplasmic antibodies (ANCAs) and various cytokines. Clinically, vasculitis may present as urticaria, livedo reticularis, purpuric papules, nodules, haemorrhagic bullae or ulcers.

Classification of vasculitis

Small vessel
- Cutaneous small vessel vasculitis (leukocytoclastic vasculitis)
- Henoch–Schönlein purpura
- Drug-induced vasculitis
- Urticarial vasculitis

Larger vessel
- Polyarteritis nodosa
- Wegener's granulomatosis
- Nodular vasculitis
- Temporal arteritis

Clinical presentations of vasculitis

Small vessel

Cutaneous small vessel vasculitis (leukocytoclastic vasculitis)

This is the most common type of vasculitis encountered in dermatology. Typically, the patient presents with numerous palpable, purpuric lesions on the legs, predominantly below the knees (Fig. 16.4). Some lesions may develop into haemorrhagic vesicles or bullae.

Histologically, there is fibrinoid necrosis of small blood vessels, and a perivascular infiltrate composed predominantly of neutrophil polymorphs. The perivascular tissues also contain extravasated red cells, and fragments of polymorph nuclei (nuclear dust). These changes are initiated by deposition of immune complexes in small vessels, complement activation and production of polymorph chemotactic factors. Polymorphs attracted to the area release enzymes that damage the vessel wall. Drugs, or bacterial or viral infections may act as the antigenic triggering factor, but often the initiating factor is not discovered.

There may be associated systemic involvement, affecting joints, kidneys and the gastrointestinal system.

Treatment. If a trigger can be identified, then it should be eliminated. A period of bed rest may result in complete resolution of the skin lesions.

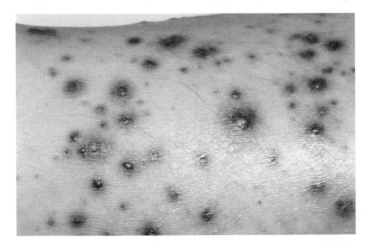

Figure 16.4 Small vessel vasculitis.

Colchicine and dapsone may be of benefit in some cases. If there is evidence of systemic involvement, treatment with systemic corticosteroids or immunosuppressive agents is required.

Henoch–Schönlein purpura (HSP)

Henoch–Schönlein purpura (anaphylactoid purpura) is the name given to a systemic small vessel vasculitis that occurs predominantly in children and is associated with deposition of IgA immune complexes in the skin (palpable purpura on elbows, knees and buttocks), joints (arthritis), kidneys (glomerulonephritis) and gastrointestinal tract (abdominal pain and gastrointestinal haemorrhage).

Upper respiratory tract infections often precede HSP.

Drug-induced vasculitis

Many drugs can be responsible for vasculitis, often of immune complex-mediated leukocytoclastic type, but other patterns occur (see Chapter 21).

Urticarial vasculitis

The appearance is similar to that of urticaria but differs in that individual lesions last longer than 24 h and often have a purpuric component. Although it is associated with a number of disorders, it is a particular feature of connective tissue diseases, predominantly Sjögren's syndrome and systemic lupus erythematusas (SLE).

Larger vessel

Polyarteritis nodosa (PAN)

Also known as periarteritis nodosa, this is an uncommon type of necrotizing vasculitis that affects medium-sized arteries throughout the body. Patients with PAN often have underlying infection with organisms that include hepatitis B and C viruses. Manifestations include pyrexia, weight loss, arthralgia and myalgia. The most significant clinical sign is the presence of cutaneous or subcutaneous nodules along the course of superficial arteries. Vessel damage results in aneurysm formation. Livedo reticularis and skin ulceration

are other features. There may be renal, gut, cardiac and nervous system involvement.

There is a type of polyarteritis nodosa that affects the skin alone. Livedo reticularis and cutaneous nodules occur on the legs, usually below the knees.

Treatment. Polyarteritis nodosa is treated with systemic steroids and immunosuppressive drugs. Purely cutaneous polyarteritis usually responds to small doses of systemic steroids.

Wegener's granulomatosis

This is a rare form of necrotizing granulomatous vasculitis affecting principally arteries of the respiratory tract, and associated with glomerulonephritis. Skin lesions take the form of a nodular vasculitis, sometimes with ulceration. It is associated with the presence of ANCAs.

Nodular vasculitis

The antigenic trigger for this form of vasculitis, which occurs predominantly in middle-aged women, is probably a bacterial infection of some type, but in many cases the precise aetiology is not discovered. Inflammatory nodules, produced by a granulomatous vasculitis in the deep dermis and subcutaneous fat, occur on the legs. These may ulcerate. Other organs are not involved.

Temporal arteritis (giant cell arteritis)

Skin changes are rare, but ulceration may occur on the temporal and parietal regions of the scalp.

Other disorders involving blood vessels

Erythema nodosum

This condition usually affects children and young adults, and is characterized by the development of multiple tender, erythematous nodules, usually on the shins (Fig. 16.5), but occasionally also on the forearms. As each nodule regresses, it changes colour from red to purple to yellow-green—like a fading bruise. Pathologically, erythema nodosum is an inflammatory process of fat (panniculitis) associated with a lymphocytic vasculitis.

Causes of erythema nodosum include:

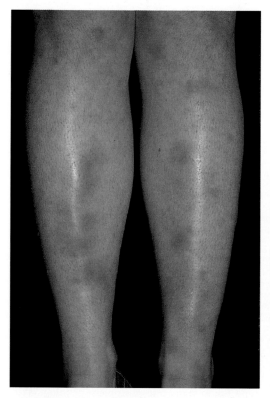

Figure 16.5 Erythema nodosum.

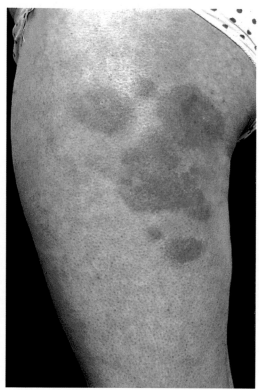

Figure 16.6 Chilblains on the thigh in a keen horsewoman.

Causes

- Streptococcal infection
- Drugs, particularly sulfonamides
- Sarcoidosis
- Primary tuberculosis
- Inflammatory bowel disease

In some cases no precipitating factor is discovered

Investigation of a patient suffering from erythema nodosum should include culture of a throat swab, antistreptolysin titre, chest X-ray and tuberculin skin test.

Treatment. In most cases bed rest and simple analgesia is all that is required. The lesions will gradually resolve over a period of a few days.

Behçet's disease

The principal features of this disorder are recurrent, severe oral and genital ulceration, and uveitis. Skin lesions include erythema nodosum and pustules at sites of minor trauma such as venepuncture sites.

Pyoderma gangrenosum (see Chapter 19)

Perniosis (chilblains)

Chilblains are painful, inflammatory lesions provoked by exposure to cold. The most common sites for chilblains are the fingers and toes, but they may also occur on fatty prominences such as the fat pads on the medial aspects of the knees, and on the thighs. A characteristic type of chilblains occurs on the lateral aspects of the thighs of female horse riders (Fig. 16.6)—this is related to the chill factor produced by galloping along in the middle of winter. 'Chilblains' is a rather unimpressive word, so dermatologists call this disorder 'equestrian cold panniculitis'.

Treatment for chilblains is not very satisfactory. The best management is prophylaxis, by wearing warm gloves and thick socks, and, in the case of the equestrian, thermal underwear and clothing made of modern insulating materials.

Chapter 17

Connective tissue disorders

Lupus erythematosus

Lupus erythematosus is an autoimmune disorder that occurs in two main forms—systemic lupus erythematosus (SLE), which affects both the skin and internal organs, and discoid lupus erythematosus (DLE), in which the skin alone is affected. A small proportion of patients suffering from DLE may subsequently develop SLE. A third variant, subacute cutaneous lupus erythematosus (SCLE), is characterized by distinctive skin lesions that may be associated with systemic features.

Systemic lupus erythematosus

This is a multisystem disorder that may affect the skin, joints, heart and pericardium, lungs, kidneys, brain and haemopoietic system. Typically, the disease affects women, particularly of childbearing age, and progresses in a series of exacerbations and remissions. Its pathogenesis is unclear, but probably involves a combination of genetic factors predisposing to autoimmunity, and environmental agents such as viral and bacterial antigens.

Mucocutaneous lesions include oropharyngeal ulceration, diffuse alopecia, Raynaud's phenomenon and photosensitivity. Often there is facial erythema in a 'butterfly' distribution (Fig. 17.1). The 'butterfly' is represented by erythema on the cheeks linked by a band of erythema across the nose. **However, by far the most common** cause of this pattern of facial erythema is rosacea.

Systemic manifestations include the following:

> **Manifestations of SLE**
>
> **Polyserositis**
> - Arthralgia and arthritis (usually non-erosive)
> - Pericarditis
> - Pleurisy with effusions
>
> **Nephritis**
> **Central nervous system involvement**
> - Psychosis and convulsions
>
> **Haemopoietic abnormalities**
> - Haemolytic anaemia
> - Leukopenia
> - Thrombocytopenia
>
> **Pyrexia, weight loss and general malaise**

Investigations

A number of autoantibodies may be found in individuals with SLE. Antinuclear antibodies (ANAs) at high titre are found in most patients with SLE, and anti-double-stranded DNA antibodies (anti-dsDNAs) are characteristic. Others include anti-Ro (also known as anti-SSA) and anti-La (anti-SSB), which are associated with neonatal lupus, and antiphospholipid antibodies. A positive rheumatoid factor and biological false-positive serological tests for syphilis may also be found.

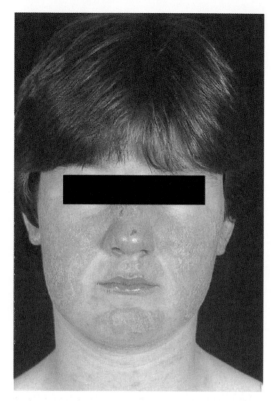

Figure 17.1 Facial erythema in systemic lupus erythematosus.

Direct immunofluorescence of skin shows a band of granular deposits of immunoglobulin G (IgG) or immunoglobulin M (IgM) at the dermo-epidermal junction.

Treatment

Systemic steroids and immunosuppressive agents are the mainstay of treatment. Light-exposed areas of skin should be protected by sun-screens with a high sun protection factor (SPF).

Antiphospholipid syndrome

This syndrome may be primary (Hughes' syndrome) or occur with SLE. The main features are the occurrence of recurrent miscarriage, venous thromboses, cerebral infarcts, thrombocytopenia and livedo reticularis. These clinical abnormalities are associated with the presence of anticardiolipin antibodies and lupus anticoagulant (subsets of antiphospholipid antibodies).

Neonatal lupus erythematosus

Neonatal lupus is associated with transplacental passage of maternal anti-Ro and anti-La antibodies. Its features include skin lesions, thrombocytopenia, hepatosplenomegaly and complete heart block. Heart block persists, but the other features resolve as maternal antibodies disappear from the infant's blood.

Drug-induced systemic lupus erythematosus

Drug-induced SLE is uncommon. The drugs most frequently implicated in its provocation include hydralazine, procainamide, anticonvulsants (phenytoin, primidone), isoniazid and chlorpromazine.

Discoid lupus erythematosus

Classically, DLE affects light-exposed areas—principally the face and neck, but also the dorsa of the hands and the arms. Lesions may be precipitated or exacerbated by sunlight. Individual lesions consist of scaling, erythematous plaques, with prominent follicular plugging. If the scale is lifted off, follicular plugs may be seen on its undersurface—the so-called 'carpet-tack' (or 'tin-tack') sign. There may be only a few lesions, but extensive, cosmetically disfiguring involvement of the facial skin can occur. Lesions heal with scarring, and the typical picture is of an active, erythematous scaly margin enclosing a central area of scarred, hypopigmented, atrophic skin (Fig. 17.2). The scalp may be involved, producing areas of scarring alopecia in which follicles are permanently destroyed. Occasionally, the buccal or nasal mucosae are affected.

Investigations

The diagnosis can be confirmed by skin biopsy. Histology shows a periadnexal lymphocytic

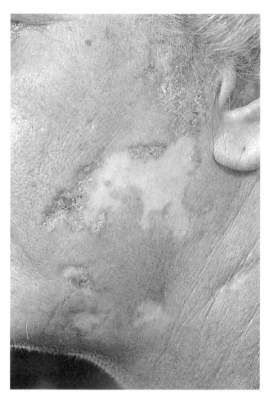

Figure 17.2 Discoid lupus erythematosus.

infiltrate, liquefaction degeneration of the basal layer of the epidermis, follicular plugging and hyperkeratosis. Direct immunofluorescence of lesional skin reveals the same pattern of immunoglobulin deposition seen in SLE (see above).

Treatment

Potent fluorinated topical steroids are helpful in many cases but, if they are ineffective, intralesional injection of triamcinolone, or oral therapy with the antimalarial hydroxychloroquine may be required. Light-exposed areas should be protected by a sun-screen with a high SPF. Where there is extensive involvement of facial skin, the use of cosmetic camouflage can be of benefit.

Subacute cutaneous lupus erythematosus

Non-scarring, papulosquamous or annular lesions occur predominantly on light-exposed areas. Associated systemic features may occur, but are usually mild.

Dermatomyositis

Heliotrope
A flower resembling the pale violet,
Which, with the Sun, though rooted-fast, doth move
And, being changed, yet changeth not her love
(Ovid)

Dermatomyositis is an autoimmune inflammatory disease of skin and muscle that may occur in childhood or in adult life. There are differences in the manifestations of the disease in these two age groups. Vasculitis and the late development of calcinosis are features of the childhood disease that are not seen in adults. In some adults, dermatomyositis is associated with systemic malignancy, whereas there is no association with malignancy in the childhood disease.

Skin

The skin changes are as follows:

Skin changes in dermatomyositis

• Violaceous erythema of the face and V-area of the neck (Fig. 17.3). This is said to resemble the colour of the heliotrope flower, and is referred to as 'heliotrope erythema'
• Periorbital oedema
• Erythema on the dorsa of the hands, and linear erythema on the dorsa of the fingers (Fig. 17.4). Erythematous papules (Gottron's papules) over the knuckles
• Prominent, ragged cuticles and dilated capillaries in the proximal nail folds (Fig. 17.5)
• Erythema over knees and elbows
• In childhood, cutaneous vasculitis leads to ulceration of the skin, particularly in the axillae and groins

---

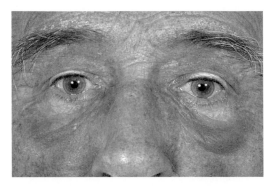

Figure 17.3 Facial erythema and periorbital oedema in dermatomyositis.

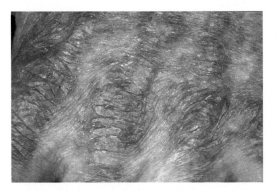

Figure 17.4 Linear erythema on the dorsa of the hands in dermatomyositis.

Muscles

In some cases, there is little evidence of any muscle disease, whereas in others there is profound muscle weakness. Typically, there is proximal, symmetrical weakness and wasting of the limb girdle muscles. Pharyngeal and oesophageal muscles may also be involved, leading to dysphagia.

Other features include pulmonary fibrosis, and arthralgia and/or arthritis.

The reported frequency of malignancy in association with adult dermatomyositis varies widely between series of patients studied, but the incidence seems to be higher in older individuals. The preferred approach to investigation appears to be performance of limited screening, in the form of careful history, thorough physical examination (rectal, lymph node, breast and pelvic examinations), full blood count, stool occult blood, cervical smear and chest radiograph. In female patients, CT or MRI scanning of the ovaries is advisable. Further investigations should be carried out in anyone with specific symptomatology.

Investigations

These include skin biopsy, serum levels of muscle enzymes, 24-h urine creatine level,

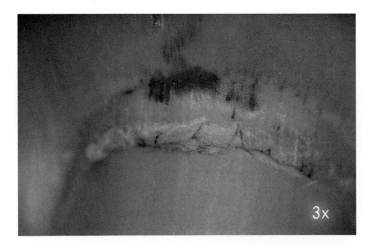

Figure 17.5 Hypertrophic cuticle, and nail fold telangiectasia in dermatomyositis.

electromyography, muscle biopsy, and ultrasound and MRI of muscles.

Treatment

In dermatomyositis associated with malignancy, there is usually marked improvement when the neoplasm is excised. A relapse of the dermatomyositis signals a recurrence.

The mainstay of therapy is oral corticosteroids. If the response to steroids is poor, immunosuppressives such as azathioprine, methotrexate or cyclophosphamide may be of benefit. Where there is severe muscle involvement, physiotherapy is an important adjunct to drug therapy, in order to minimize contractures.

Scleroderma

Scleroderma means 'thickening of the skin', and is a term applied to a group of diseases in which there is sclerosis of the skin and destruction of hair follicles and sweat glands. Scleroderma may be an isolated cutaneous phenomenon, when it is called 'morphoea', or a cutaneous component of a multisystem disorder.

Morphoea

This is a disorder of unknown aetiology in which there is sclerosis of the skin. It may be subdivided clinically into the following types:

1 Circumscribed.
2 Linear.
3 Frontoparietal (*en coup de sabre*).
4 Generalized.

Circumscribed

This is the most common clinical presentation of morphoea. Solitary or multiple indurated plaques develop, predominantly on the trunk. Initially, affected areas of skin have a violaceous hue, but gradually become thickened and ivory in colour (Fig. 17.6). The surface is smooth and shiny. Eventually, usually after many months, the sclerosis resolves, leaving atrophic, hyperpigmented areas.

Classification of scleroderma

• Morphoea: sclerosis of the skin without systemic involvement
• Systemic sclerosis: cutaneous sclerosis in association with a vasculopathy of small arteries producing multi-organ systemic disease
• Chemically induced scleroderma: sclerosis of the skin as a manifestation of the toxic effects of certain chemicals
• Pseudoscleroderma: sclerosis of the skin associated with a number of diseases other than morphoea or systemic sclerosis

---

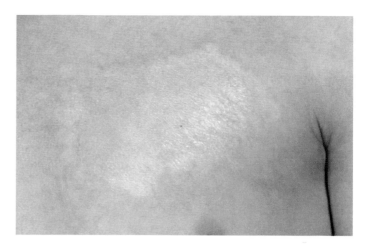

Figure 17.6 A plaque of morphoea.

Linear

Linear morphoea usually affects one limb, often extending its full length. In childhood, it can significantly impair the growth of the limb, and produce severe flexion deformities of large joints and digits.

Frontoparietal (*en coup de sabre*)

Resembling a sabre cut across the scalp and forehead, this type of morphoea is a considerable cosmetic problem. A linear, depressed, sclerotic area extends from the face into the scalp, and is associated with loss of hair along its length.

Generalized

There is extensive sclerosis of the skin on the trunk and limbs. Flexion contractures restrict limb movement, and if the chest is severely affected breathing may be impaired.

Treatment

There is no effective treatment for morphoea. In linear morphoea on the limbs, physiotherapy is essential to maintain joint motility, and orthopaedic surgery may be necessary. Plastic surgery can be of considerable cosmetic benefit in frontoparietal morphoea.

The natural history of morphoea is gradual spontaneous resolution.

Systemic sclerosis

The pathogenesis of systemic sclerosis is unknown. It is a disorder in which sclerotic changes in the skin occur as one component of a multisystem disorder associated with a vasculopathy of small arteries. In the most common form (sometimes referred to as the CREST syndrome (Calcinosis, Raynaud's phenomenon, (o)Esophageal involvement, Sclerodactyly and Telangiectasia)), skin changes affect predominantly the face and hands.

Systemic involvement

Gastrointestinal. Dysphagia is the result of oesophageal involvement. Damage to the myenteric plexus leads to hypomotility of smooth muscle and later to atrophy and fibrosis, resulting in impaired peristalsis. The gastro-oesophageal sphincter mechanism is also impaired, leading to gastro-oesophageal reflux, oesophagitis and eventual stricture formation. Symptoms of oesophageal reflux are common.

Atrophy and fibrosis of the smooth muscle of the small bowel lead to impaired peristalsis, and the resultant relative stagnation of small-bowel contents predisposes to bacterial overgrowth as colonic bacteria move upstream into the small intestine. Gut bacteria deconjugate bile salts (which are essential for micelle formation) and this leads to fat malabsorption and steatorrhoea. Occasionally, patients present with a picture simulating acute intestinal obstruction.

Similar pathology affects the large bowel and leads to the formation of multiple wide-mouthed pseudodiverticula.

Pulmonary. An inflammatory alveolitis is followed by pulmonary fibrosis, and disease of small pulmonary arteries leads to pulmonary hypertension and cor pulmonale.

Cutaneous features of systemic sclerosis

Face
• The facial skin is sclerotic and bound to underlying structures, producing a tight, shiny appearance, with loss of facial wrinkles, a beaked nose, and restriction of mouth opening (Fig. 17.7)
• Perioral furrowing ('purse-string mouth')
• Facial telangiectasia
• Loss of lip vermilion

Hands
• Raynaud's phenomenon
• Tight sclerotic skin producing progressive contractures of the digits (sclerodactyly)
• Finger pulp infarcts producing small, painful ulcers (Fig. 17.8). These infarctive changes lead to progressive pulp atrophy and resorption of the underlying terminal phalanges
• Calcinosis (Fig. 17.9)

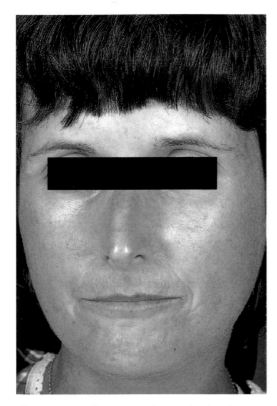

Figure 17.7 Facial appearance in systemic sclerosis.

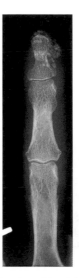

Figure 17.9 X-ray showing calcinosis in a digit in systemic sclerosis.

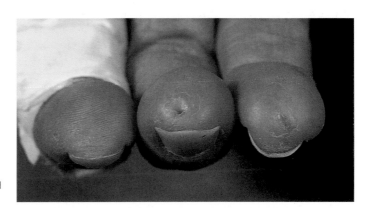

Figure 17.8 Finger pulp ulcers and scars in systemic sclerosis.

Renal. Fibrinoid changes in arteries and arterioles are associated with proteinuria and hypertension. Renal involvement is usually mild, but in some cases it is severe and rapidly progressive, and leads to renal failure.

Nervous system. Neurological involvement is uncommon, but carpal tunnel syndrome and trigeminal neuropathy have been reported.

Cardiac. Myocardial fibrosis, conduction disorders and a variety of electrocardiographic (ECG) abnormalities have been described.

Hepatic. There is a significant association between systemic sclerosis and primary biliary cirrhosis.

Musculoskeletal. Arthralgia and arthritis occur in some patients, and myopathy and inflammatory myositis may also occur.

Treatment

No therapy is known to alter the overall course of systemic sclerosis, but many components of the disease may be helped significantly by specific measures. Digital ischaemia may be helped by electrically heated gloves and socks. Calcium-channel blockers may help relieve Raynaud's phenomenon. Patients with oesophageal reflux should avoid lying flat, and treatment with proton-pump in-hibitors may be very effective. Broad-spectrum antibiotics are helpful in treating patients with gut bacterial overgrowth and malabsorption.

Prognosis

Severe pulmonary or renal involvement are poor prognostic factors, but most patients suffering from systemic sclerosis live for many years.

Chemically induced scleroderma

Polyvinyl chloride (PVC) can induce a disorder resembling idiopathic systemic sclerosis, and 'vinyl chloride disease' has been described in workers in the PVC industry, particularly reactor cleaners. A number of other chemicals may induce diseases mimicking systemic sclerosis, including perchlorethylene and trichlorethylene (solvents used in dry cleaning), and bleomycin. A disorder similar to systemic sclerosis occurred in 1981 in people poisoned by contaminated rape-seed oil sold as cooking oil in Madrid.

Pseudoscleroderma

Scleroderma-like changes may be seen in a number of unrelated conditions, including porphyria cutanea tarda, carcinoid syndrome and phenylketonuria.

Chapter 18

Pruritus

There was a young belle of old Natchez
Whose garments were always in patches
When comment arose
On the state of her clothes
She drawled: 'When ah itchez, ah scratchez!'
(Ogden Nash, *Requiem*)

Pruritus means itching. *Please* note the correct spelling: it is *not* spelt *pruritis*, as often appears in student examination papers, clinical notes and referral letters!

Pruritus varies in duration, localization and severity. Everyone has experienced short-term, localized, itch, and there is a perverse joy in having a really good scratch. However, some individuals suffer from distressing chronic irritation lasting for years. Itching may be restricted to one or more sites, or cover virtually the whole body surface. It may creep about, appearing first on an arm and later on the back, or in more than one site simultaneously. Itching can be mild or appallingly severe, constant and distressing. Chronic pruritus can completely ruin the quality of life.

Pruritus is prominent in many skin diseases. Especially itchy are the eczemas, lichen planus, insect bites and infestations, urticaria and dermatitis herpetiformis. However, the skin may also itch when there is no rash.

Mechanisms of pruritus

We do not clearly understand why skin diseases itch, and we know very little about irritation in otherwise apparently normal skin.

The sensation that we call itch is produced, conditioned and appreciated at several levels in the nervous system: stimulus; mediators and receptors; peripheral pathways; central processing; interpretation. A wide variety of stimuli can induce an itch, and a number of chemicals may be involved, especially histamine, prostaglandins and some proteinases. However, the details remain obscure: although histamine can induce itch without wealing, non-sedative antihistamines have no effect on simple pruritus.

More complex, central mechanisms may also be important in modulating and appreciating pruritus. Many itch-provoking stimuli induce pain if applied at higher intensities. Indeed, scratching appears to induce pain and to abolish irritation. However, other sensory stimuli can also abolish itching, and more complex mechanisms have been proposed. One theory involves a complicated filtering system controlling input pathways to further stimuli and passing information on to higher centres.

Itching can certainly be affected by higher centres. It is much less apparent when the mind is fully occupied and much worse when boredom sets in. 'Stress' and other psychological factors can induce or worsen pruritus.

Causes of pruritus

The term 'pruritus', used without qualification, implies that there is itching without a *primary* skin disorder. However, in many instances there are considerable *secondary* skin changes from scratching (e.g. excoriations, scars and prurigo—see below).

But watch out! Subtle changes are easily obscured by scratching: a classical example of this is scabies (see Chapter 5). A full history and a careful examination of the skin are therefore important in all patients complaining of itching.

In considering causes, we shall look separately at localized itching, generalized states and so-called 'senile' pruritus.

Localized pruritus

Localized irritation of the skin is common. The skin may be normal, but it is more common to find some abnormalities.

Two very important and troublesome forms of localized pruritus are lichen simplex chronicus and prurigo, and anogenital pruritus.

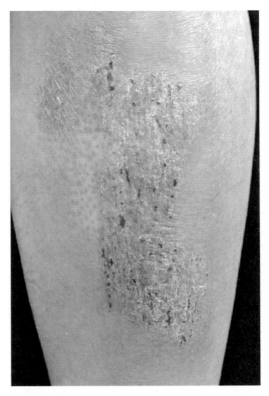

Figure 18.1 Lichen simplex chronicus.

Lichen simplex chronicus and prurigo

This difficult problem is sometimes called 'neuro-dermatitis'. Constant irritation leads to constant scratching which, in turn, leads to thickening of the skin. This may occur in plaques, known as lichen simplex chronicus (Fig. 18.1), or in nodules, which are given the name *prurigo* (Fig. 18.2). The areas are intensely irritable, and a self-perpetuating itch/scratch cycle develops. Patients who develop this kind of localized itching are often rather tense.

Sites of predilection. Cassical sites for lichen simplex chronicus—include shins, forearms, palms and the back of the neck (sometimes known as 'lichen nuchae'); perianal and vulval skin may also be affected (see below). Prurigo nodules may accompany areas of lichen simplex or appear separately almost anywhere; they are frequently multiple.

Lesions are often asymmetrical.

Treatment. Potent topical steroids (sometimes under occlusive bandages) may help, but the problem often recurs.

Anogenital pruritus

Two very common (and least talked about) forms of localized itching are pruritus vulvae and pruritus ani. They may be encountered together.

Pruritus ani is often attributed to haemorrhoids. However, although haemorrhoids and tags are often present, their treatment alone does not always relieve the symptoms. The problem is also often dismissed as psychological, but only rarely is this the complete explanation.

Anal itching may continue for years. Irritation is often spasmodic and extremely intense. The majority of patients are male.

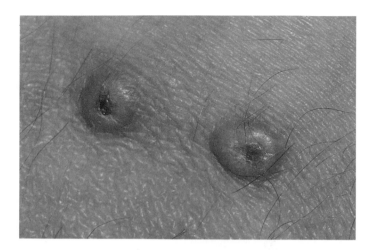

Figure 18.2 Nodular prurigo.

Clinical features. Examination often reveals little abnormality; there may be some excoriation and thickening of anal and perianal skin; 'tags' are often present; occasionally gross changes amounting to lichen simplex are seen; there may be an associated fissure.

Aetiology. Pruritus ani is probably largely a low-grade irritant reaction to faeces, sweat and discharge; sedentary occupations make matters worse. Contact allergy to medicaments may be a factor, especially allergy to local anaesthetics and preservatives. Psoriasis of the natal cleft and perineum may give rise to pruritus ani.

Pruritus vulvae can be very distressing. There are a number of causes to consider.

Treatment depends upon the cause.

Treatment of perineal irritation

'Irritant' pruritus ani
• Good hygiene, a high fibre diet and treatment with topical steroids are useful
• Treating concomitant haemorrhoids may reduce discharge

Skin disorder and allergic contact dermatitis
• Most will require topical steroids

Candidosis
• Antifungal creams and pessaries; check for diabetes

No changes seen
• Patients seldom respond to antipruritics
• Inexpert psychological probing is valueless

Causes of pruritus vulvae

• Mild incontinence (with prolapse) may cause irritant changes
• Skin disorders: notably eczema, psoriasis and lichen sclerosus (et atrophicus) (see Chapter 15)
• Allergic contact dermatitis to medicaments (as in anal itch — see above)
• Candidosis (secondary to diabetes): the vulva is beefy red, and there may be pustules and a vaginal discharge
• Vulval itch with no visible signs, when a true psychogenic origin is suspected

Generalized pruritus

Generalized pruritus is extremely unpleasant, and can either affect most of the body surface continuously or involve several different areas. By definition, a primary skin disorder has been excluded.

Clinical features. Skin changes vary considerably—nothing to see at all; mild flakiness of the skin, with a few scratch marks; or the skin may be covered in excoriations, scars and nodules. The skin is often dry, especially in elderly patients.

Although there may be no identifiable underlying disorder, all patients with generalized irritation should be investigated because a number of potentially remediable systemic disorders may be responsible.

Systemic disorders causing irritation

Haematological disorders
- Iron deficiency
- Polycythaemia rubra vera

Cholestatic liver disease
- Extrahepatic obstruction
- Primary biliary cirrhosis
- Hepatitis
- Drug-induced cholestasis

Chronic renal failure
Thyroid disease
- Thyrotoxicosis
- Myxoedema

Malignancy
- Lymphomas and leukaemias
- Carcinomas

Drug ingestion
- Especially opiates

Pregnancy (see Chapter 15)

Haematological disorders

Chronic iron deficiency may be due to blood loss (e.g. from menorrhagia or a gut carcinoma). Many elderly patients and some vegans are iron deficient for dietary reasons. Polycythaemia rubra vera is characteristically associated with itching triggered by bathing.

Liver disease

The itch is probably related to bile salts in the skin. Irritation may precede the development of other features of cholestatic liver disease, especially in primary biliary cirrhosis.

Chronic renal failure

Unfortunately the intractable itch is largely unaffected by dialysis. Parathyroidectomy is said to help, but the benefit is short-lived and is hardly justified in most patients.

Thyroid disease

Both thyrotoxicosis and myxoedema may present with pruritus. In myxoedema the general dryness of the skin may be responsible.

Cancers

Lymphoreticular malignancies are particularly prone to cause itching, but pruritus may also occur in association with a variety of carcinomas. Up to 30% of Hodgkin's disease patients suffer from generalized pruritus.

Drugs

Various agents induce itching, but the mechanisms are poorly understood. Opiates appear to act centrally and on mast cells. Oestrogens and phenothiazines induce cholestasis.

Diabetes mellitus

You may come across lists quoting diabetes as a cause of itching, but we do not consider that this is the case.

Psychological factors

When everything else has been excluded, psychological factors may be considered. The most common underlying problem is an anxiety neurosis, but patients with monodelusional psychoses such as parasitophobia also itch. These individuals, however, offer their own explanation only too readily! (see Chapter 20).

Screening procedures for generalized pruritus are as follows:

Screening for generalized pruritus

- A full history and general examination
- Full blood count
- ESR (or plasma viscosity)
- Liver function tests
- Blood urea/urea nitrogen/creatinine
- Iron studies
- Serum thyroxine
- Urine protein
- Chest X-ray

If these tests are negative initially, and if the pruritus persists, repeat at intervals

---

Treatment

Treatment of generalized pruritus is that of its cause. When no apparent underlying reason can be found, a topical steroid and a sedative antihistamine, such as hydroxyzine, may help. Some authorities recommend opiate antagonists and UVB phototherapy.

'Senile' pruritus

Itching with no apparent cause is common in elderly people. It may be mild and localized, but can be very severe and generalized. The patients (and their carers) are often anxious and miserable, but this is usually secondary to the irritation rather than a primary cause. This state is called 'senile pruritus'. It is not known what causes ageing skin to itch.

Examination

The skin is texturally either 'normal' or 'dry'. Excoriations, secondary eczematization and areas of infection are common. Localized areas of 'eczema craquelé' may develop (see Chapter 7).

Treatment

Treatment is extremely difficult. Sedative antihistamines often cause excessive drowsiness and confusion, and topical steroids are of limited use. If the skin is texturally 'dry', liberal use of emollients may be helpful. Care has to be taken, however, as these agents can make both the patient and their surroundings very slippery!

Increased frequency of washing or the use of harsh soaps and detergents makes matters worse, both by removing surface lipids and by acting as direct irritants. Soaps should therefore be used sparingly and emollients employed instead.

Chapter 19

Systemic disease and the skin

The skin may be involved directly or indirectly in a number of systemic disease processes, and can provide visible diagnostic clues which could lead to the discovery of internal disease.

Endocrine disease

Diabetes

There are a number of cutaneous manifestations of diabetes, including the following:

Cutaneous features of diabetes

1 Certain cutaneous infections
2 Neuropathic ulcers
3 Necrobiosis lipoidica
4 Diabetic dermopathy
5 Diabetic bullae
6 Xanthomas
7 Acanthosis nigricans
8 Lipoatrophy
9 Cheiroarthropathy

---

1 Cutaneous infection. Mucosal candidiasis, particularly balanitis and vulvovaginitis, and carbuncles, occur more frequently in diabetics.
2 Neuropathic ulcers. Impaired sensation, as a result of sensory neuropathy, predisposes to the development of neuropathic ulcers on the soles of the feet (Fig. 19.1).

3 Necrobiosis lipoidica. Lesions of necrobiosis lipoidica characteristically occur on the shins, although they may develop elsewhere. The lesions are initially erythematous, but subsequently become yellowish-brown and atrophic, and underlying blood vessels are easily seen through the thinned skin (Fig. 19.2). Occasionally the lesions ulcerate. Good diabetic control does not appear to influence the skin lesions.

Potent topical steroids and intralesional steroid injections are among several treatments suggested for necrobiosis lipoidica, but results of therapy are not very impressive.
4 Diabetic dermopathy. This term is applied to small, brown, scar-like lesions seen on the shins in some diabetics. The lesions are thought to be associated with diabetic microangiopathy.
5 Diabetic bullae. In this uncommon blistering disorder of diabetics, subepidermal bullae occur on the hands and feet. Their aetiology is unknown.
6 Xanthomas. Hyperlipidaemia in uncontrolled diabetes may be associated with the development of multiple small, yellow, eruptive xanthomas.
7 Acanthosis nigricans. In association with insulin resistance.
8 Lipoatrophy. Insulin-resistant diabetes associated with partial or generalized cutaneous lipoatrophy.
9 Cheiroarthropathy. A scleroderma-like thickening of the skin of the hands in insulin-dependent diabetics.

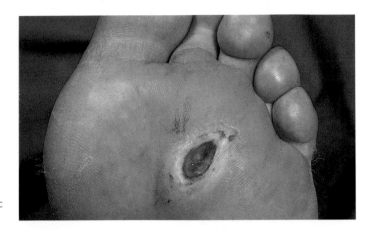

Figure 19.1 Diabetic neuropathic ulcer.

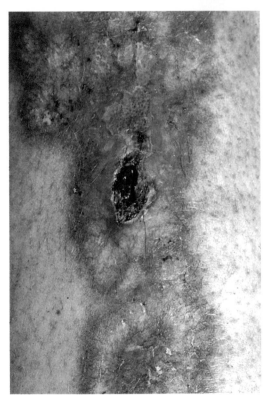

Figure 19.2 Necrobiosis lipoidica with a small ulcerated area.

Granuloma annulare

There is no significant association between classical granuloma annulare and diabetes, but in a much rarer, generalized form of granuloma annulare there is an association with diabetes. Typically, lesions of granuloma annulare are groups of firm, skin-coloured papules, often arranged in rings, and commonly occurring on the dorsa of the hands and feet (Fig. 19.3). The natural history of granuloma annulare is eventual spontaneous resolution, but persistent lesions may be treated with intralesional triamcinolone or cryotherapy.

Thyroid disease

Hypothyroidism

The skin is typically dry, and feels thickened due to subcutaneous mucin deposition—hence the designation myxoedema. A malar flush on an otherwise pale face produces what has been referred to as a 'strawberries and cream' appearance. There may be a yellowish tinge to the skin, said to be due to the deposition of carotenes. There is often periorbital oedema. Scalp hair is diffusely thinned and there is loss of the outer part of the eyebrows. Sitting close to the fire to keep warm may produce severe erythema ab igne ('granny's tartan') on the shins, but since the advent of central heating this physical sign has become uncommon.

Hyperthyroidism

Cutaneous changes that may accompany thyrotoxicosis include excessive sweating, palmar erythema, diffuse alopecia, generalized hyperpigmentation and thyrotoxic acropachy (digital clubbing). The nails may show onycholysis. Some patients develop pretibial myxoedema,

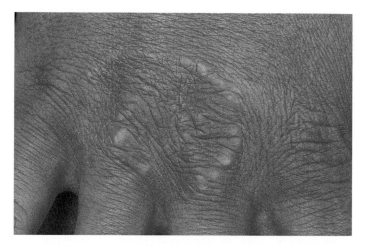

Figure 19.3 Granuloma annulare.

which is produced by subcutaneous deposition of excessive amounts of mucopolysaccharide, and is characterized by erythema and thickening of the soft tissues over the shins and dorsa of the feet.

Vitiligo may accompany autoimmune thyroid disease, and generalized pruritus may be a feature of both hypo- and hyperthyroidism.

Adrenal disease

Cushing's syndrome

The cutaneous effects of Cushing's syndrome include thinning of the skin, spontaneous bruising, prominent striae on the trunk and limbs, diffuse alopecia, acne and hirsutism.

Addison's disease

Diffuse hyperpigmentation is the main cutaneous manifestation of Addison's disease. The pigmentation is particularly prominent on the buccal mucosa and in the palmar creases. Vitiligo may also accompany autoimmune Addison's disease.

Rheumatic diseases

Gout

In addition to tophaceous deposits around affected joints, gouty tophi may occur on the ears.

Still's disease

This is a disorder of childhood, although it may rarely occur in adults. Accompanying the pyrexial episodes of Still's disease is a diffuse maculopapular eruption that characteristically develops in the late afternoon and evening, and usually resolves by the following morning. Some slander-mongers claim that dermatologists never see this eruption because its periodicity is outside their normal working day!

Rheumatoid arthritis

Dermatological features include the following:

> **Dermatological features of rheumatoid arthritis**
>
> • Rheumatoid nodules. Subcutaneous nodules over bony prominences, particularly on the extensor aspect of the forearms and the dorsa of the hands
> • Vasculitic lesions. Digital vasculitis may produce small infarcts around the nail folds (Bywaters' lesions), or more severe digital ulceration and even gangrene. Vasculitic lesions may also occur on the legs, and contribute to the development of leg ulcers
> • Pyoderma gangrenosum (Fig. 19.4)
> • Palmar erythema

Rheumatic fever

Almost extinct in developed countries, rheumatic

fever may be accompanied by a characteristic eruption, erythema marginatum.

Reiter's syndrome

Predominantly a disease of young adult males, Reiter's syndrome is a reactive arthropathy usually precipitated by non-specific urethritis, but occasionally by bacillary dysentery. In addition to urethritis, conjunctivitis/uveitis and arthritis, there may be an eruption which is indistinguishable from psoriasis. On the soles of the feet the skin lesions may become extremely thickened, producing so-called 'keratoderma blennorrhagicum'. The buccal mucosa may show scattered erosions, and superficial circumferential erosive changes on the penis are referred to as 'circinate balanitis'.

Vitamin deficiency

Scurvy

The classical picture of vitamin C (ascorbic acid) deficiency is rarely seen nowadays in developed countries, but scurvy may be encountered in elderly people and in alcoholics, as a result of nutritional self-neglect. The typical appearance is of perifollicular purpura, easy bruising, poor wound healing and bleeding gums.

Pellagra

Pellagra is the result of nicotinic acid deficiency. Classically, it has three major manifestations—dermatitis, diarrhoea and dementia. The dermatitis affects light-exposed areas, and there is often a well-demarcated margin to the affected area on the neck (Casal's necklace). Pellagra may occur in alcoholics as a result of nutritional self-neglect, and in food faddists. A similar dermatitis may be provoked by isoniazid in individuals who are slow acetylators of this drug.

Hyperlipidaemia

Both primary and secondary hyperlipidaemic states may be associated with lipid deposits in the

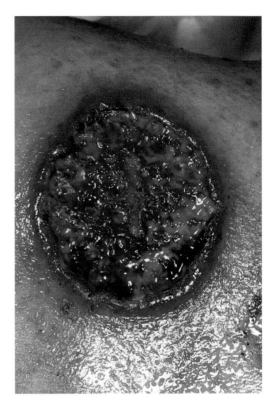

Figure 19.4 Pyoderma gangrenosum.

skin, known as xanthomas. There are several different clinical types of xanthomas. Orange-yellow lipid deposits in the eyelid skin are known as xanthelasma (Fig. 19.5). Tuberous xanthomas occur as yellowish nodules, usually over bony prominences (Fig. 19.6). Tendinous xanthomas, as their name suggests, are deposits of lipid in association with tendons, often involving the Achilles tendons and extensor tendons on the dorsa of the hands. Deposits of lipid in the skin creases of the palms of the hands (striate palmar xanthomas) appear to be particularly associated with primary type III hyperlipidaemia (broad beta disease; dysbetalipoproteinaemia). Eruptive xanthomas are crops of yellowish papules that occur in association with marked hypertriglyceridaemia.

Inflammatory bowel disease

Ulcerative colitis and Crohn's disease may be

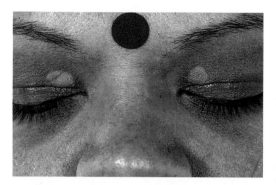

Figure 19.5 Xanthelasma.

associated with a number of mucocutaneous manifestations including the following:

Mucocutaneous features of inflammatory bowel disease

• Pyoderma gangrenosum. The lesions may be single or multiple. They initially resemble boils, which subsequently break down to form necrotic ulcers with undermined purple edges (Fig. 19.4). Pyoderma gangrenosum may also occur in association with rheumatoid arthritis, myeloma and leukaemia. The treatment of choice is systemic steroids, but azathioprine, minocycline, clofazimine and ciclosporin (cyclosporin) may also be effective
• Erythema nodosum
• Perianal and buccal mucosal lesions. In Crohn's disease, anal examination may reveal fleshy tags, fissures and perianal fistulae. The buccal mucosa may be oedematous and ulcerated, and the lips may be swollen as a result of a granulomatous cheilitis

---

Amyloidosis

In systemic amyloidosis, amyloid deposits in the tongue produce macroglossia, and cutaneous deposits are visible as yellowish, waxy, purpuric plaques around the eyes and in the perianal area.

Sarcoidosis

Sarcoidosis is a multisystem granulomatous disorder of unknown aetiology. There are a number of patterns of skin involvement, including the following:

Skin patterns in sarcoidosis

• Erythema nodosum. Tender, erythematous nodules on the legs (see Chapter 16)
• Lupus pernio. The skin of the nose and ears is involved in the granulomatous process, and becomes swollen and purplish in colour
• Scar sarcoid. Sarcoid granulomas localize in old scar tissue, making the scars prominent
• Papules, nodules and plaques. These often have an orange-brown colour

---

Liver disease and the skin

Changes in the skin and nails which occur in association with chronic liver disease include the following:

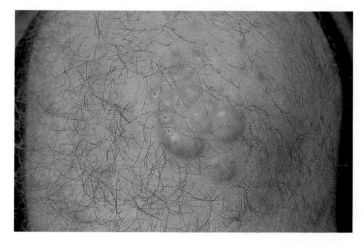

Figure 19.6 Tuberous xanthomas.

Skin and nail changes in liver disease

- Palmar erythema
- Pruritus: in cholestatic liver disease
- Spider naevi: in a superior vena caval distribution
- Xanthelasma: in primary biliary cirrhosis
- White nails (Terry's nails)
- Pigmentary changes: in addition to jaundice, patients with longstanding cholestatic liver disease may also have marked melanin pigmentation. Patients suffering from haemochromatosis have generalized bronze-brown pigmentation that is produced by a combination of iron and melanin

Cutaneous manifestations of systemic malignancy

Cutaneous metastases

Malignant tumours may metastasize to the skin, and tumours of renal, ovarian, gastrointestinal, breast and bronchial origin are those most likely to do so. Cutaneous metastases usually present as pink nodules, and occur most frequently on the scalp and anterior trunk. Scalp metastases may produce areas of alopecia (alopecia neoplastica).

Lymphatic extension of carcinoma to the skin may produce an area of erythematous induration resembling cellulitis, and known as 'carcinoma erysipeloides'.

Metastasis of ovarian or gastrointestinal carcinoma via the ligamentum teres can present as an umbilical nodule (Sister Joseph's nodule).

Miscellaneous cutaneous signs of underlying malignancy

1 **Dermatomyositis** (see Chapter 17).
2 **Acanthosis nigricans.** This is a warty, hyperpigmented thickening of skin in the flexures (Fig. 19.7). The palms of the hands may also be affected, producing an appearance known as 'tripe palms'. The most common associated malignancy is an adenocarcinoma of the gastrointestinal tract. However, 'malignant' acanthosis nigricans is rare.
3 **Generalized pruritus.** Generalized itching, without a rash, may be associated with a wide variety of systemic malignancies.

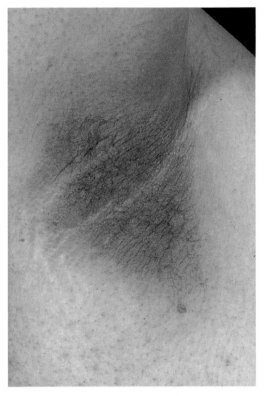

Figure 19.7 Acanthosis nigricans.

4 **Thrombophlebitis migrans.** This is particularly associated with carcinoma of the pancreas.
5 **Acquired ichthyosis.** Ichthyosis developing for the first time in adult life may be associated with a lymphoma.
6 **Pyoderma gangrenosum.** This may occur with myeloma and leukaemia.
7 **Necrolytic migratory erythema.** This is a distinctive eruption associated with pancreatic glucagonoma.
8 **Flushing** and a rosacea-like eruption are cutaneous features of the carcinoid syndrome.
9 **Erythema gyratum repens.** This rare skin marker of malignancy is a bizarre eruption whose appearance resembles wood grain.
10 **Acquired hypertrichosis lanuginosa.** The sudden growth of profuse vellus hair over the face and body is a rare sign of underlying neoplastic disease.

11 Paraneoplastic pemphigus. This rare blistering disorder typically occurs in patients with lymphoproliferative diseases.

Leukaemia and the skin

There are numerous cutaneous changes that may accompany leukaemia, or be provoked by the drugs used in its treatment.

Common presenting features of acute leukaemia include purpura, bruising, and bleeding from the gums, and the skin may be directly involved in the form of leukaemic infiltrates. Disseminated herpes zoster (herpes zoster with numerous outlying vesicles) may accompany leukaemia, as may a severe bullous form of pyoderma gangrenosum, and Sweet's disease (acute febrile neutrophilic dermatosis).

Purpura

Purpura is produced by extravasation of red cells into the skin, and has numerous causes. The lesions do not blanch on pressure.

Causes of purpura include vasculitis (see Chapter 16), quantitative or qualitative platelet abnormalities, drugs, amyloidosis, dysproteinaemias and infections (e.g. meningococcaemia).

AIDS and the skin

Patients with AIDS are at increased risk of developing a number of mucocutaneous problems:
1 Oral candidiasis extending into the oesophagus.
2 Oral 'hairy leukoplakia'—white ridges along the sides of the tongue, caused by Epstein–Barr virus.
3 Seborrhoeic dermatitis: this is often severe, and is probably related to an altered host response to *Malassezia* yeasts.
4 Papular pruritic eruption and eosinophilic folliculitis are manifest as itchy papular lesions and are signs of advanced immunosuppression. They are probably part of the same spectrum. Their aetiology is unknown.
5 Staphylococcal infection, shingles, molluscum contagiosum and dermatophyte fungal infection occur more commonly in AIDS patients.
6 Episodes of herpes simplex are more frequent and more severe, and lesions may become chronic.
7 Perianal warts tend to be more florid and more difficult to treat.
8 Kaposi's sarcoma: a tumour which is thought to arise from vascular endothelium and is related to infection with human herpesvirus type 8 (HHV-8) infection. Lesions are usually multiple, and may affect any part of the skin, as well as internal organs. It is rarely the cause of death in AIDS patients, who usually succumb to intercurrent infection. It is a radiosensitive tumour.
9 Pre-existing psoriasis may become severe and extensive in AIDS patients.
10 Bacillary angiomatosis. Caused by the bacillus *Bartonella henselae*, these angioma-like lesions affect the skin, mucosae and internal organs. They respond to treatment with erythromycin.
11 Drug-associated problems. The antiretroviral treatment now widely employed in treating HIV infection may provoke rashes and cause nail pigmentation. In addition, a cosmetically troublesome lipodystrophy, characterized by symmetrical loss of subcutaneous fat, which on the face produces a cachectic appearance, is associated with highly active antiretroviral therapy (HAART).

Chapter 20

Skin and the psyche

If you happen to have a wart on your nose or fore-head, you cannot help imagining that no one in the world has anything else to do but stare at your wart, laugh at it, and condemn you for it, even though you have discovered America. (Fyodor Dostoevsky, *The Idiot*)

Patients with skin disease who often ask 'Is it caused by nerves, doctor?' are usually trying to es-tablish if they can attribute their skin condition to 'stress'. In fact, few skin disorders are directly relat-ed to psychological disturbance. However, there is evidence that psoriasis and atopic eczema may be exacerbated by stress, and other conditions in which emotional stress has been claimed to play a part in some cases include alopecia areata and acute pompholyx.

There is no doubt that skin disease has psycho-logical effects on the patient, and can significantly adversely affect their quality of life. Skin disease is visible to others, it carries the taint of contagion, and affected individuals often feel stigmatized and have poor self-image and low self-esteem. They will be aware that their skin is being scrutinized, and that any form of physical contact, such as shaking hands or collecting change, may provoke apprehension in others. In ethnic groups where marriages are arranged, the presence of skin disease may compromise marriage prospects, and cause considerable emotional distress.

Infections with ectoparasites sometimes have marked psychological effects. Patients feel un-clean, and these feelings can persist long after the problem has been eradicated.

There are some skin disorders which are directly related to psychological problems, and these are described below.

Dermatitis artefacta

Patients with dermatitis artefacta produce skin le-sions to satisfy a psychological need, but what ben-efit they derive from their actions is usually not obvious. There is no rational motive for their be-haviour. If challenged, they will vehemently deny that the lesions are self-induced. As a group they are distinct from malingerers, who consciously im-itate or produce an illness for a deliberate end.

Dermatitis artefacta is more common in women, and most of those affected are adolescents or young adults. However, there is a subgroup with an older age of onset who are more likely to be male. Many have some connection with the health pro-fessions, either directly or via family members.

Artefactual skin lesions may be produced in a number of different ways including rubbing, scratching, picking, gouging, puncturing, cutting, sucking, biting, the application of heat or caustics, or the injection of milk, blood or faecal material. Limb oedema may be simulated by the intermit-tent application of constricting bands (Secretan's syndrome). Lesions tend to have bizarre geometric shapes that do not conform to those seen in naturally occurring disease—no dermatosis has square, rectangular or triangular lesions. Often the lesions are more numerous on the side of the body opposite the dominant hand. If a caustic material such as an acid has been used to induce lesions, this may trickle off the main area of damage to produce the 'drip-sign' of tell-tale streaks at the margins. Even when suspected artefactual lesions are covered with occlusive dressings, patients will often manage to insert knitting needles under the dressings, or push sharp instruments through them, in order to continue damaging the skin.

The history obtained from these patients is devoid of any useful information about the evolution of their lesions. The impression conveyed is that one minute the skin was normal, and the next it was blemished. This so-called 'hollow history' is characteristic, as is a striking complacency about what are often extremely disfiguring lesions ('*la belle indifference*'), sometimes accompanied by an enigmatic 'Mona Lisa' smile. One patient we have seen, who had extensive suppuration of the left arm, probably produced by the inoculation of faeces (Fig. 20.1), said about her arm 'Yes, it is rather unpleasant isn't it. I wonder if you could arrange for someone to take it off'.

When they see the severity of the lesions and an apparent lack of progress in diagnosis and treatment, relatives and friends of the patient quite naturally rally to their support, and may be somewhat vocal in their criticism of a seemingly inept medical profession. Other doctors caring for the patient may also be convinced that their disease is naturally occurring. This situation, in which other individuals 'support' a patient with dermatitis artefacta, is known as '*folie à deux*', and is also encountered in delusions of parasitosis (see below).

The psychopathology of patients who produce artefactual lesions is not uniform, but in some cases there is a demonstrable personality disorder, and in others significant depression.

It requires considerable expertise to be able to make a confident diagnosis of dermatitis artefacta, but even experienced dermatologists see cases in which they suspect the lesions are self-induced, but cannot be certain. Alternatively, there are occasional cases in which there is a strong suspicion of dermatitis artefacta, but the lesions are discovered to be the result of naturally occurring disease.

Treatment is extremely difficult in many cases. Confronting the patient with the diagnosis achieves very little, in that it usually produces a categorical denial that they are producing the lesions, and subsequent failure to attend for follow-up. Strict occlusion of the traumatized areas may allow healing, but the lesions will reappear as soon as occlusive dressings are removed. An alarming consequence of occlusion may be the appearance of lesions elsewhere, or the development of other

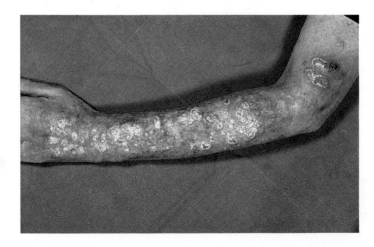

Figure 20.1 Dermatitis artefacta—in this case probably the result of inoculation of faeces into the skin.

'symptoms', as if to compensate for inability to reach the usual sites. Antidepressants will help those who are depressed. Psychiatric referral is often unhelpful and, unfortunately, many patients refuse assistance from a psychiatrist. The situation often remains at stalemate. As long as the doctor's suspicions are not voiced, the patient appears content to continue attending for follow-up.

The course of this disorder is often protracted. Recovery often has little to do with successful medical treatment, but occurs because of increasing maturity, marriage or having children.

Dermatological pathomimicry

Dermatological pathomimicry is distinct from dermatitis artefacta. Patients with this condition either deliberately perpetuate their skin disease, or reproduce a pre-existing skin disorder. Having been appraised of the aetiology of their skin disease, they use this knowledge to reproduce the lesions when under emotional stress, to obtain sympathy, or in an effort to avoid an unpleasant situation with which they cannot cope. Examples of the type of illness used by patients for pathomimicry include allergic contact dermatitis, drug reactions and chronic leg ulceration.

Sympathetic discussion with the patient will usually solve the problem.

Dermatological non-disease (dysmorphophobia)

In this condition, patients complain of severe symptomatology localized to certain parts of the body, most commonly the face, scalp and perineum, but without any objective evidence of disease. The complaints include dysaesthesias such as burning, itching or throbbing pain; too much or too little hair on the face or scalp, or altered texture of scalp hair; and the belief that they are the source of an offensive odour, usually from the axillae or feet. These delusional beliefs or perceptions of abnormal sensations are a consuming preoccupation for the patient. Perineal symptoms in men include complaints of a red, burning scrotum, and the female equivalent is a burning discomfort in the vulva (vulvodynia). There is nothing abnormal to see on examination.

In some cases, depression is part of the picture; others may be suffering from monosymptomatic hypochondriacal psychosis. There is a significant risk of suicide. Management is difficult, but some patients respond to treatment with antidepressants and psychotherapy.

Delusions of parasitosis (parasitophobia)

The individual with delusions of parasitosis has an unshakeable conviction that their skin is infested with parasites. An experienced dermatologist will recognize this disorder from information supplied in the referral letter, and will often arrange to see the patient at the end of a clinic, because the consultation is usually extremely lengthy. However, before seeing a dermatologist, the patient has often consulted their local university department of zoology or a medical entomologist in an attempt to identify the 'parasites'. They will also probably be known to companies specializing in pest eradication, who will have been asked to disinfest their home. They may have isolated themselves from family and friends because of their fear of passing the 'infestation' on to them and, because of their absolute conviction that they are infected, they may have convinced their family, friends and even the family doctor of the reality of the problem (shared delusion; *folie à deux*).

Patients often describe a feeling of itching, biting or 'crawling' in the skin (formication), and state that when this occurs they are able to remove a small 'insect' or 'worm' from a skin 'lesion'. When asked to demonstrate typical skin 'lesions', they will often point to Campbell de Morgan spots, freckles or other minor blemishes. Typical 'specimens' are presented to the doctor wrapped in pieces of paper or adhesive tape, and kept in a matchbox (Fig. 20.2). These should always be examined under the microscope, because they just might contain parasites, but usually they contain fragments of cotton or skin debris.

It is impossible to persuade these patients that parasites are not responsible for their condition. If they are shown that their 'specimens' are simple debris they remain unconvinced, and may even suggest that the parasites are so small that an electron microscope will be required to demonstrate them. In this situation, the most lucid, eloquent discourse will fall upon deaf ears—the patient's beliefs remain unshaken, and the doctor usually retires from the conflict feeling more than somewhat jaded.

Delusions of parasitosis may occur in association with organic brain disease such as senile dementia and cerebral arteriosclerosis, and has been described in pellagra, vitamin B_{12} deficiency and following coronary bypass surgery. The term 'monosymptomatic hypochondriacal psychosis'

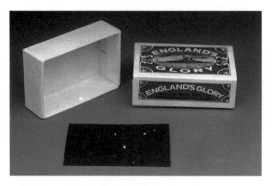

Figure 20.2 Matchbox and 'specimens' in delusions of parasitosis.

may be applied to patients with a single, fixed delusion, and most patients with delusions of parasitosis fit into this category.

Effective treatment is very difficult, and many patients continue with their delusion for years. As with dermatitis artefacta, a confrontational approach rarely achieves anything. Patients often refuse psychiatric help because they do not accept that they have a mental illness, and cannot see how a psychiatrist could possibly help with what, to them, is a physical disorder. The neuroleptic drug pimozide, or the newer antipsychotic risperidone, may be of benefit.

Obsessive–compulsive habits

Trichotillomania

Trichotillomania means compulsive plucking of hair. The scalp is involved most often, but the eyebrows and eyelashes may be affected. A mild form of trichotillomania may be observed in libraries, where engrossed students compulsively twist locks of hair around their fingers, but they rarely pull it out unless examinations are approaching! The clinical picture is of patches of hair loss containing hairs of varying length. Often the crown of the head is affected, and the hair at the margins is of normal length (Fig. 20.3). The underlying scalp is usually normal, but may be excoriated.

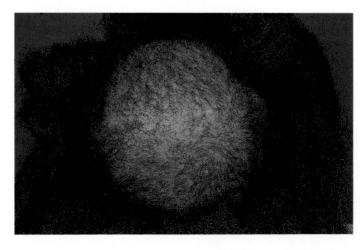

Figure 20.3 Trichotillomania.

Trichotillomania in childhood is often transient. However, it may be a manifestation of significant psychopathology, particularly in adults.

Neurotic excoriations

This disorder is encountered predominantly in middle-aged women. The lesions are produced by picking and gouging, and are usually scattered over the arms, upper trunk and face. More recent lesions are usually interspersed with scars from previous excoriations. Acne excoriée is a variant of this condition in which minimal acne lesions are repeatedly picked and gouged, leaving scars when the lesions heal.

Patients with this problem have obsessive–compulsive personalities, and picking the skin appears to provide relief of unconscious aggression and tension. Antidepressants and supportive psychotherapy may be of benefit.

Chapter 21

Cutaneous drug reactions

There are only two types of drug—those that don't work and those that have side-effects. (Bruno Handel FRCS)

Introduction

The skin is one of the most common sites for unwanted drug effects (a better term than 'side-effects'), although estimates of the frequency vary considerably. Cutaneous drug reactions are probably under-reported and certainly often go unrecognized. Note, though, that skin disorders wholly unrelated to drug ingestion can be labelled erroneously. It is important not to jump to conclusions: we have seen viral infections and scabies diagnosed as drug reactions. There are many people who state they are 'allergic to penicillin', but who are not.

Cutaneous drug reactions may be due to several different mechanisms. Unfortunately there are no reliable *in vitro* tests for establishing that a rash is due to a drug. Simple *in vivo* tests, such as prick testing and patch testing, have a limited place in specific situations, but usually yield no useful information either. However, even if the mechanism(s) for a particular reaction is known (and it often isn't), a test may not be appropriate because the reaction is not to the drug itself, but to a drug complex or metabolite that is produced *in vivo* after ingestion or administration.

The only definitive test is direct challenge with the suspected agent, but this may be impossible or unethical in many circumstances. For these reasons, proving that a specific eruption was due to a specific drug is difficult, and judgements usually have to be made on clinical grounds alone.

Causes of drug reactions
• Simple intolerance
• Hypersensitivity: types I, II, III and IV
• Pharmacokinetic disturbances
• Drug interactions
• Complex interactions between host, drug and environment (e.g. light)

Drug reaction patterns

However, all is not lost! Some drugs are much more prone to induce cutaneous drug reaction patterns than others. Common offenders include:

Drugs causing skin reactions
• Antibiotics (especially penicillin, semisynthetic penicillins and sulfonamides)
• Non-steroidal anti-inflammatory drugs
• Hypnotics
• Tranquillizers

Furthermore, there are a number of well-defined clinical drug reaction patterns. Some of these patterns are more specific to certain drugs, and this may help to identify the culprit.

Common cutaneous drug reaction patterns

- Exanthematic eruptions
- Urticaria and anaphylaxis
- Exfoliative dermatitis
- Vasculitis
- Fixed drug eruptions
- Lichen planus-like eruptions
- Erythema multiforme
- Acneiform eruptions
- Hair abnormalities
- Pigmentary changes
- Bullous reactions
- Photosensitivity
- Lupus erythematosus-like syndrome
- Exacerbation of pre-existing skin disease

Exanthematic eruptions

The most common cutaneous drug reactions are itchy, widespread, symmetrical, erythematous and maculopapular (Fig. 21.1): there is often a strong resemblance to a viral exanthem. The time relationship is variable: in most instances the rash begins a few days after starting the drug, but it may begin almost immediately, or be delayed for a few weeks. Exanthematic eruptions usually fade a week or so after stopping the drug, but exfoliative dermatitis may develop (see below and Chapter 15).

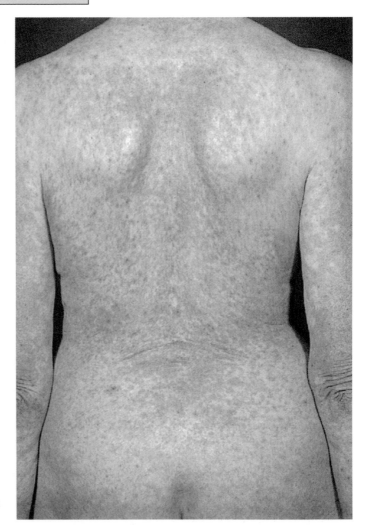

Figure 21.1 A typical exanthematic eruption due to an antibiotic.

Common causes. Non-steroidal anti-inflammatory drugs and antibiotics, particularly ampicillin, other semisynthetic penicillins, sulfonamides and gentamicin.

Rarer causes. Gold, barbiturates and phenothiazines.

Urticaria and anaphylaxis (see also Chapter 15)

Drug-induced urticaria may be due to a direct pharmacological action on mast cells, or to type I or type III hypersensitivity reactions.

Occasionally, drugs may trigger a major anaphylactic reaction, with or without urticaria, which can be fatal unless treated very rapidly. Unfortunately, there is no known way of predicting this disaster.

Common causes. Aspirin, opiates (direct), penicillins, cephalosporins, pollen vaccines and toxoids (immune).

Eczema

Type IV hypersensitivity reactions to topical medicaments are common, and give rise to a contact dermatitis (see Chapter 7). Figure 21.2 shows a man who was given eye drops containing an aminoglycoside. Occasionally, a topically sensitized patient may receive the compound (or a closely related chemical) systemically. The result is a severe, widespread, eczematous reaction.

Common causes. Lanolin in creams and bandages; preservatives (parabens, ethylenediamine) in creams; topical anaesthetics (*not* lidocaine (lignocaine)); topical antihistamines; topical antibiotics, especially aminoglycosides, in creams and drops; increasingly, topical steroids.

Exfoliative dermatitis

Drugs are one of the four important causes of exfoliative dermatitis (see Chapter 15).

Common causes. Prominent offenders are sulfonamides and sulfonylureas, gold, phenytoin, allopurinol and barbiturates.

Vasculitis (see Chapter 16)

Drug ingestion is a common trigger for vasculitis.

Common causes. Thiazides, captopril, cimetidine, quinidine, sulfonamides.

Fixed drug eruptions

Fixed drug eruptions are one of the most curious events encountered in dermatological practice.

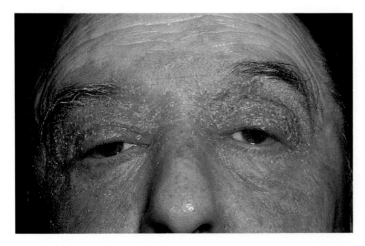

Figure 21.2 Contact sensitivity to neomycin.

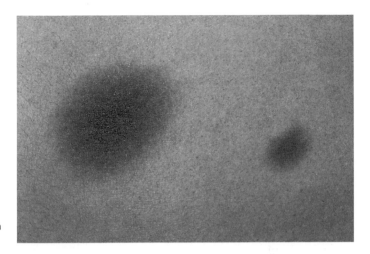

Figure 21.3 Fixed drug reaction to a sulfonamide.

The reaction occurs in the same place(s) every time the offending drug is taken. They are often misdiagnosed as recurrent eczema or ringworm.

A round or oval patch of dusky erythema develops, often with a purplish centre (Fig. 21.3), and sometimes a central bulla. This fades to leave postinflammatory hyperpigmentation. There may be only one lesion or multiple sites. Fixed eruptions can occur anywhere, but the limbs and genitalia are favoured sites.

Common causes. Laxatives containing phenolphthalein, sulfonamides, dapsone, tetracyclines, barbiturates.

Lichen planus-like eruptions

Lichen planus-like (sometimes known as 'lichenoid') reactions are rare, but can be severe. The eruption is occasionally indistinguishable from idiopathic lichen planus, but more commonly there is an eczematous element, with much more scaling. In severe cases, an exfoliative dermatitis may develop (see above and Chapter 15).

Causes. Antimalarial drugs; some beta-blockers; sulfonylureas; gold. Thiazides may cause lichen planus-like eruptions on light-exposed surfaces.

Erythema multiforme (see Chapter 15)

So many things seem to be able to trigger erythema multiforme that it is usually difficult to be certain whether a drug is responsible.

Suggested drug causes. Barbiturates; long-acting sulfonamides; cotrimoxazole; rifampicin.

Acneiform eruptions

Skin changes resembling acne vulgaris occur with several drugs. The changes tend to be monomorphic, consisting largely of papulopustules. There are seldom comedones present.

Causes. Corticosteroids (both topical and systemic), adrenocorticotrophic hormone (ACTH), androgenic drugs, lithium and iodides. Some drugs also exacerbate pre-existing acne (see below).

Hair abnormalities

As discussed in Chapter 13, drugs may be responsible for hair loss or excessive hair growth.

Pigmentary changes

Several drugs cause pigmentary changes (Table 21.1).

Table 21.1 Drugs causing cutaneous pigmentary changes.

Colour	Drug
Characteristic generalized reddish-brown hue	Clofazimine (used in leprosy)
Yellow	Mepacrine
	Carotene
Purplish	Chlorpromazine
Blue–black	Chloroquine (especially on shins)
	Minocycline (in high dosage)
	Amiodarone (on light-exposed sites)
Brown	Oestrogens (= chloasma)

Heavy metals such as silver may be deposited in the skin following industrial exposure or ingestion (e.g. in antismoking lozenges).

Bullous reactions

There are several ways in which drugs may induce blistering.

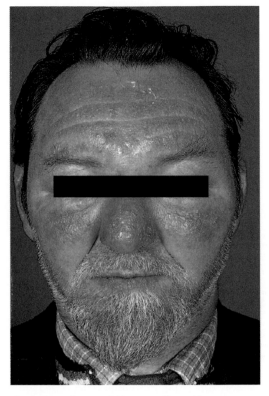

Figure 21.4 Photosensitivity to a sulfonamide.

Drug-induced blistering

- In fixed drug eruptions
- Drugs may induce pemphigus and pemphigoid (see Chapter 14)
- Drugs may exacerbate porphyria cutanea tarda
- Nalidixic acid may cause a dramatic phototoxic bullous reaction
- Barbiturates may be associated with bullae on bony prominences, usually in patients unconscious due to overdose

---

Photosensitivity

There are three main types of reaction.

Photosensitive reactions

- Exacerbation of underlying disease
- Direct phototoxic reaction
- Photoallergic reaction

In phototoxic reactions, the dose of the drug and the intensity of ultraviolet exposure may both be important: if critical levels are not reached, the reaction may not develop. This can be confusing if the drug has been taken on a number of occasions.

Patients complain that exposure to the sun causes a burning sensation followed by erythema, swelling and, later, eczematous changes on light-exposed areas (Fig. 21.4).

Common causes. Phenothiazines; sulfonamides; tetracyclines; thiazides. Demethylchlortetracycline can cause photo-onycholysis. Bullae due to nalidixic acid have been mentioned above.

Lupus erythematosus-like syndrome

A rare but important drug reaction is the induction of a syndrome closely resembling systemic lupus erythematosus.

Causes. Many agents have been incriminated, including hydralazine, isoniazid, penicillin, minocycline, procainamide and griseofulvin.

Exacerbation of pre-existing disease

Some drugs may produce a deterioration in certain skin disorders. Notable examples are:

1 Acne—androgenic drugs (e.g. danazol, stanozolol), oral contraceptives and corticosteroids.

2 Porphyrias—all clinical features, including cutaneous photosensitivity, may be worsened by drug ingestion, particularly barbiturates and oestrogens.

3 Psoriasis—lithium, antimalarials.

4 Systemic lupus erythematosus—penicillin and sulfonamides may produce deterioration.

Conclusion

If you use all the clinical information at your disposal, it is often possible to determine if a rash is drug provoked, and what the causitive agent might be.

Clinical information

- A good history
- A careful examination
- Elimination of other skin diseases
- Recognition of the clinical reaction pattern
- Matching the reaction with the most likely offender

and

- Tests, where appropriate (possibly including a challenge)

Chapter 22

Treatment of skin disease

If it's dry, wet it. If it's wet, dry it. Congratulations, you are now a dermatologist! (Anonymous)

The above witticism is oft-quoted by non-dermatologists as an assessment of the scope of dermatological therapeutics. An alternative calumny relates to a dermatologist murmuring an unintelligible Latin name as a diagnosis and then prescribing a topical steroid, for everything. Apart from being deeply offensive to sensitive skin doctors, both these quips are far from the truth, as dermatologists have an enormous therapeutic armamentarium at their disposal. In days of yore, it must be admitted, many of the available topical therapies resembled witches' brews containing 'Eye of newt and toe of frog, wool of bat and tongue of dog'. They were often cosmetically unacceptable and malodorous—if the skin disease did not render the patient a social pariah, the treatment could be relied upon to do so. However, in recent years, topical therapies have become not only more effective, but also cosmetically much more acceptable.

The treatment of individual disorders has been dealt with in preceding chapters, and this chapter is designed to provide an overview of the principles of therapy.

Topical therapy

An ideal topical preparation for the management of skin disease would penetrate well, but remain lo-calized within the skin, thereby avoiding potential problems from systemic effects. In practice, this is extremely difficult to achieve, and any agent that penetrates the stratum corneum is absorbed to some extent.

Topical preparations consist of an *active ingredient* (or ingredients) and a material in which this is suspended—a *base*. These components must be compatible. There is little point in discovering a new base that penetrates the skin like a hot knife through butter if it completely inactivates everything suspended in it.

The stratum corneum forms a natural protective barrier to penetration of externally applied agents. Hence, to facilitate penetration by a drug, this barrier function must be breached, and this can be achieved by hydration of the stratum corneum—for example, penetration of a topical steroid may be markedly enhanced by occluding an area of skin with polythene. Unfortunately, if large areas of skin are occluded in this way, the amount of steroid absorbed may be sufficient to produce systemic effects. Bases containing urea also hydrate the stratum corneum and enhance penetration of their active ingredients. Dimethyl sulfoxide (DMSO) is a solvent that penetrates skin extremely rapidly, and is used as a vehicle for the antiviral agent idoxuridine.

Bases

Bases include creams, oily creams, ointments, lotions, gels and pastes. A *cream* is an oil-in-water emulsion that is relatively non-greasy and has only limited emollient activity. Creams are cosmetically acceptable and can be used to treat either moist or dry skin conditions. *Oily creams* are water-in-oil emulsions which combine good emollient properties with cosmetic acceptability and are therefore of benefit in dry skin conditions. *Ointments* are greasy preparations that have emollient and occlusive properties. The occlusive effect of an ointment results in hydration of the stratum corneum and enhanced penetration of the active ingredient of the ointment. The benefits of ointments are offset by a lack of cosmetic acceptability. Ointments are messy and stick to clothing. If used on the hands they transfer to everything touched—an obvious disadvantage to someone employed in clerical work, for example. *Lotions* are fluid preparations that have a cooling effect due to evaporation. They are useful in the management of moist, exudative skin lesions, and also in dermatoses affecting the scalp. Clear, non-greasy *gels* are designed for use on hairy parts of the body, where they are cosmetically acceptable. *Pastes* are powders, usually mixed with soft paraffin, and are protective—for example, in the prevention of maceration of the skin around a discharging ulcer.

The choice of a particular base should be determined by the type of skin problem and the sites affected. It is, for example, wholly inappropriate to prescribe a steroid ointment for daytime use on the scalp, because it is too messy. A gel or lotion preparation should be used instead. Similarly, a lotion is not the correct base for ichthyotic skin, where an oily cream or ointment are more appropriate.

Bases are mixtures of several components, formulated to provide stability and freedom from microbial contamination. Random dilution of a topical preparation will dilute the preservatives in the base and significantly shorten its shelf-life.

Communication and patient compliance

Most non-topical medication involves popping pills of various colours into the mouth at certain times of the day, requiring a minimum of effort and only a minor feat of memory. Topical therapy demands a great deal more of the patient, and the increased effort required of the patient ought to be matched by the provision of precise instructions by the doctor. Verbal instructions are not sufficient if multiple topical therapies are prescribed. For example, a patient suffering from psoriasis might be given a tar shampoo, a steroid scalp lotion, a mild topical steroid cream to use in the flexures, and a dithranol preparation for short contact therapy to plaques on the trunk and limbs. If the patient has only recently developed psoriasis, and is not familiar with its treatment, the provision of multiple therapies without clear instructions could easily lead to confusion.

Do not expect patients who depart for work at the crack of dawn to adhere strictly to instructions to wash their hair every morning and use a topical medication twice daily. Modify the treatment schedule to suit the individual. If you are prescribing a preparation which is messy to use and/or malodorous, warn the patient about this. For example, dithranol stains and benzoyl peroxide bleaches, and lack of prior warning, could lead to ruined clothing and bed-sheets.

It is a useful exercise to imagine your own level of compliance if encumbered with a skin disease requiring regular treatment.

Quantities prescribed

It is important when prescribing topical therapy to consider the area to be covered and the frequency of application before assessing the quantity of a topical agent required by the patient. For example, there is little point in prescribing a 30-g tube of an emollient to be used over the entire body surface after bathing—this hardly constitutes a week's supply for an ichthyotic gerbil. A repeat prescription would be required after one application, because this is the approximate amount necessary for a single application over the whole body surface of an adult. Topical therapies are available in a variety of container sizes. You will need to check the available sizes before prescribing, as they vary from product to product. Topical steroids, for example, may be marketed in 15-, 25-, 30-, 50- or 100-g tubes, depending on the manufacturer and the steroid. Most emollients are available in 50- and 100-g tubes and 500-g tubs or dispensers.

Underprescribing and overprescribing are both common. One does not require 100 g of cream to treat a small patch of eczema on the leg—most of the tube will languish in a drawer or bathroom cabinet until its shelf-life is long expired, or it may be used inappropriately by another member of the family. However, someone regularly using an emollient over extensive areas of skin should be given 500-g dispensers.

Topical steroids

At first sight the huge number of available topical steroids is bewildering to the uninitiated, but with a little knowledge and experience their use is quite straightforward. They are divided into several groups according to potency. Hydrocortisone preparations are the weakest. However, hydrocortisone in a base containing urea, which enhances penetration of the stratum corneum, is moderately potent. Modification of the basic steroid skeleton by fluorination (fluorinated steroids) or esterification produces steroids of much greater potency (Table 22.1).

Choice of preparation

The most appropriate topical steroid for a given situation should be determined by the type and

Table 22.1 Steroid potency.

Potency	Examples
Mild	1% Hydrocortisone
Moderately potent	Clobetasone butyrate (Eumovate)
	Flurandrenolone (Haelan)
	Alclometasone dipropionate (Modrasone)
	Hydrocortisone with urea (Alphaderm)
Potent	Betamethasone valerate (Betnovate)
	Fluocinolone acetonide (Synalar)
	Fluocinonide (Metosyn)
	Hydrocortisone butyrate (Locoid)
Very potent	Clobetasol propionate (Dermovate)
	Diflucortolone valerate (Nerisone Forte)

severity of the condition being treated, the sites affected and the age of the patient. The skin disorders that are responsive to steroids have been delineated in previous chapters, and include various types of eczema, lichen planus, psoriasis of the scalp, flexures, hands and feet, and discoid lupus erythematosus. In general, a severe dermatosis should be treated with a potent steroid, and a mild condition with a weak steroid. In the case of a chronic dermatosis subject to periodic exacerbations, a mild to moderate potency steroid can be used when the condition is quiescent, and a potent preparation when it worsens.

There are regional variations in the absorption of topical steroids through the skin and their potential for local adverse effects. These variations are determined by the thickness of the stratum corneum; occlusion, for example in the flexures where skin surfaces are in apposition; and the vascularity of the area. Most facial dermatoses should only be treated with mild topical steroids, although a few conditions such as discoid lupus erythematosus will require potent preparations. Skin disease affecting the axillae, groins and submammary areas should also be treated with mild topical steroids. Conversely, dermatoses of the palms and soles, where the stratum corneum is extremely thick, require potent steroids, and a greater benefit is often obtained if polythene occlusion is used to enhance penetration.

There is a greater risk of adverse systemic effects from the use of topical steroids in children because of the high ratio of skin surface area to body volume, particularly in infants. For this reason, mild topical steroids should be used in small children. The skin of elderly people is thin, and potent steroids will amplify this change—their use over long periods of time should therefore be avoided or carefully supervised.

Side-effects

Side-effects are rarely seen following the use of mild topical steroids, but they are encountered more frequently in association with potent topical steroid use, although much less commonly than in the early years of steroid availability.

Case studies

Case 1

A 5-year-old boy was referred because of suspicion that skin lesions on his buttocks were the result of non-accidental injury in the form of cigarette burns. Another child in the family had been taken into care following concerns about its well-being.

Examination

There were several lesions on both buttocks, varying in size, and consisting of small pustules and large superficial erosions with crusting (Figs C1.1 and C1.2). The child was otherwise perfectly well.

What is the diagnosis?

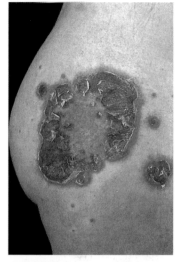

Figure C1.1

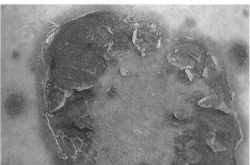

Figure C1.2

Case 2

A young woman complained of itchy, dark patches on both temples. She had a similar, but larger, patch on the abdomen.

Examination

There were symmetrical patches of hyperpigmented dermatitis on the temples (Fig. C2.1), and a large patch on her abdomen adjacent to the umbilicus.

What is the likely cause of her problem?

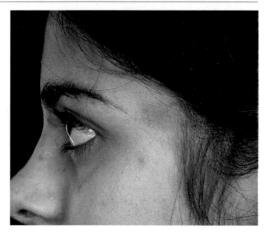

Figure C2.1

See page 192 for answers

Case 3

A 28-year-old woman had been troubled by an itchy rash on the feet for several years. She had used several topical steroid preparations with some symptomatic relief, but the rash persisted. In addition, she had noticed that her toenails were abnormally thickened and difficult to cut, and she attempted to camouflage the changes with nail varnish (Fig. C3.1).

Examination

There was extensive fine scaling on the feet, with some background redness. All the toenails were thickened, discoloured and friable.

What is the diagnosis?

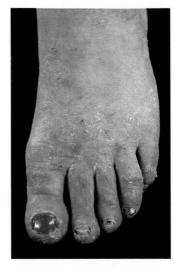

Figure C3.1

Case 4

An elderly woman in residential care has been treated for extremely itchy 'eczema' on her trunk and limbs for several months. Even the most potent topical steroids have failed to resolve the problem, and she has an extensive rash. Because several other residents have similar problems, suspicion has fallen on the biological detergent used when washing bed-linen.

Examination

She is scratching persistently and there are extensive eczematous changes on her trunk and limbs (Fig. C4.1). In addition, there are numerous lesions on her hands (Fig. C4.2) and feet. The other affected residents have similar lesions.

What is the diagnosis?

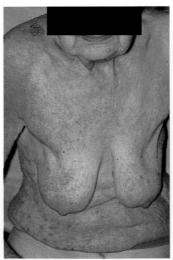

Figure C4.1

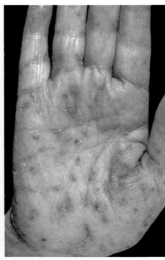

Figure C4.2

Case 5

A 57-year-old man complained of a small lump on his right ear. It had been present for about 12 months and had hardly increased in size, but was a nuisance because whenever it was touched, or if he attempted to sleep with the right side of the head on the pillow, it was extremely painful. His family doctor thought it looked like a small basal cell carcinoma. There were no other skin lesions.

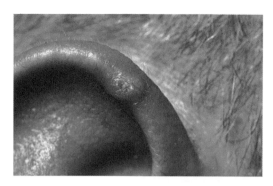

Figure C5.1

Examination

There was a papule with a central crust on the helix rim of the right ear (Fig. C5.1). When pressure was applied to the centre of the lesion it was obviously extremely painful.

What is the diagnosis?

Case 6

An 18-year-old girl developed a widespread rash affecting the trunk, limbs and scalp.

Examination

There were multiple pink, scaly patches on the trunk and limbs (Fig. C6.1), along the scalp margin and in the scalp itself. There were prominent lesions on the elbows.

What is the diagnosis?

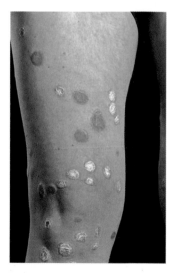

Figure C6.1

Case 7

A 6-year-old girl attended with her parents because she had developed increasing problems with a rash on the face, neck, trunk and limbs. She had been scratching all areas vigorously and had made herself bleed on occasion. She was particularly distressed at night and had not been sleeping well (nor had her parents).

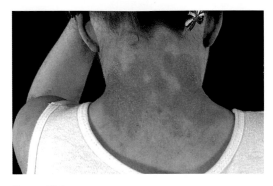

Figure C7.1

Examination

There was marked redness over both cheeks with some scaling and evidence of scratching (excoriation). The skin on the arms, legs and trunk felt dry and rough, and there was widespread, blotchy erythema, including the back of the neck (Fig. C7.1), the antecubital and popliteal fossae.

What is the diagnosis?

Case 8

A 45-year-old female lawyer was referred urgently, having noticed a pigmented mole on her left calf. She had first become aware of it about 6 months previously, but was concerned when she realized that it had enlarged since then.

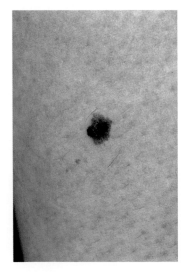

Examination

There was a darkly pigmented lesion, 2.5 × 3.5 cm, with a markedly irregular edge, on the left calf (Fig. C8.1). There was no lymphadenopathy.

What is the diagnosis?

Figure C8.1

Case 9

A 55-year-old woman presented with a 2-week history of a generalized itchy rash. She had been taking several prescription drugs for a number of years, including a beta-blocker, diuretic, angiotensin-converting enzyme (ACE) inhibitor and an oral antidiabetic agent. She finished a course of amoxicillin for a urinary tract infection 3 weeks ago.

Examination

There was a maculopapular rash affecting all parts of the body with a striking degree of symmetry (Fig. C9.1).

What is the most likely cause of her rash?

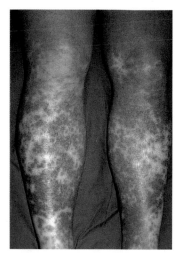

Figure C9.1

Case 10

A 76-year-old retired postmistress was referred because she had rapidly developed a severe eruption on both legs below the knees. She had a long history of problems with varicose veins and, in addition to surgery on the veins, had been treated for varicose eczema and ulceration with a variety of topical agents, including medicated bandages.

Examination

There was extensive weeping eczema on both legs below the knees (Fig. C10.1).

What is the probable reason for development of the severe eczema?

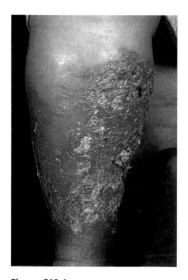

Figure C10.1

Answers to case studies

Case 1

Diagnosis

The appearance is characteristic of bullous impetigo (see Chapter 3), with pustules and superficial bullae whose roofs are quickly abraded, leaving erosions at the margins of which the stratum corneum is peeling back (Fig. C1.2). An exudate dries to form a crust. This appearance is not infrequently mistaken for burns resulting from non-accidental injury.

Case 2

Diagnosis

This is allergic contact dermatitis to nickel (see Chapter 7), related to her well-worn spectacle frames (Fig. C2.2). The patch on her abdomen was caused by contact with a jeans stud.

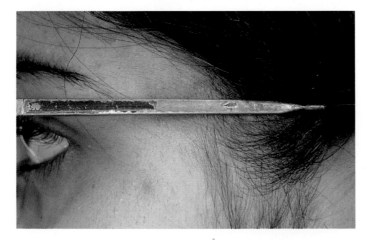

Figure C2.2

Case 3

Diagnosis

This is tinea incognito (see Chapter 4). Inappropriate use of topical steroids has suppressed the inflammatory response to the fungus, which would usually be evident on the dorsum of the foot as scaly erythema with a raised red margin to the affected area. The infection has spread inexorably to produce diffuse scaling, and infection of the toenails (onychomycosis) is responsible for their abnormal appearance.

Remember, if a rash one would expect to improve on treatment with potent topical steroids does not, always re-assess the diagnosis.

Case 4

Diagnosis

She and the other residents have scabies (see Chapter 5). The assumption that her primary problem was eczema led to inappropriate use of potent topical steroids. This, in turn, partially suppressed the immune response to the mites and was associated with reduced itching and scratching, thus allowing the mites to proliferate. Hence the large number of burrows on the hands (Fig. C4.2). In time it is likely that she would have developed crusted (Norwegian) scabies. The detergent, often blamed for dermatoses but rarely the cause, was innocent.

Case 5

Diagnosis

This is chondrodermatitis nodularis (don't bother trying to remember the rest of the name—it probably has the longest name for the tiniest lesion) in its most frequent site, i.e. the helix rim of the right ear in a man over the age of 50 (see Chapter 9). The history is absolutely typical. Its clinical features often lead to a misdiagnosis of BCC. However, it would be rare to see a BCC in this site, and if one did occur it would probably be asymptomatic when only this size.

Case 6

Diagnosis

This is psoriasis (see Chapter 8). There are small plaques with silvery scale. The presence of lesions on the elbows is also highly suggestive of psoriasis.

Case 7

Diagnosis

This is atopic eczema (dermatitis) (see Chapter 7). The problem often begins in the first few months of life, but can appear at any age. Involvement of the flexures is an important sign.

Case 8

Diagnosis

This is a thin (good prognosis) superficial spreading melanoma (see Chapter 9). The history and site are typical.

Case 9

Diagnosis

The most likely explanation is a drug eruption triggered by the antibiotic (see Chapter 21). It is always important to take a careful drug history in anyone presenting with sudden onset of a symmetrical eruption. Allergy to drugs can develop even after years of treatment, although recent additions are the most probable cause, as in this case.

Case 10

Diagnosis

It is likely that she has developed allergic contact dermatitis to a component or components of her topical medication. Patients who are being treated for varicose eczema and ulceration have often used numerous topical agents and these may contain sensitizing components such as antibiotics or preservatives. A rapid worsening and spread of varicose eczema should therefore prompt investigation by patch testing once the exacerbation has been treated.

Multiple choice questions

1. **Which of the following are potential adverse effects of potent topical corticosteroids?**
   A Perioral dermatitis
   B Hypopituitarism
   C Cushing's syndrome
   D Crusted scabies
   E Striae

2. **Physical signs in neurofibromatosis include which of the following?**
   A Crowe's sign
   B Cullen's sign
   C Darier's sign
   D Nikolsky's sign
   E Auspitz sign

3. **Which of the following diseases may be associated with pyoderma gangrenosum?**
   A Pseudomembranous colitis
   B Ulcerative colitis
   C Myeloma
   D Pancreatic glucagonoma
   E Rheumatoid arthritis

4. **Erythema multiforme may be triggered by which of the following?**
   A Herpes simplex
   B *Mycoplasma* infection
   C Orf
   D Staphylococcal infection
   E Drugs

5. **The Koebner phenomenon is a feature of which of the following diseases?**
   A Toxic epidermal necrolysis
   B Psoriasis
   C Vitiligo
   D Atopic dermatitis
   E Lichen planus

6. **Which of the following can indicate an underlying malignancy?**
   A Dermatomyositis
   B Generalized pruritus
   C Lichen planus
   D Erythema marginatum
   E Acquired ichthyosis

7. **Clothing (body) lice are responsible for transmission of which of the following diseases?**
   A Epidemic typhus
   B Lyme disease
   C Bubonic plague
   D Trypanosomiasis
   E Malaria

8. **There is a known association between crusted (Norwegian) scabies and which of the following?**
   A Erythrodermic psoriasis
   B HIV/AIDS
   C Down's syndrome
   D Darier's disease
   E Ichthyosis

9. **Which of the following are true of scabies?**
   A Itching develops 4–6 weeks after initial infection
   B Mites live in the hair follicles
   C Contact with clothing worn by an infected individual often results in transmission of the disease
   D Red papules on the penis and scrotum are an important physical sign
   E A Scandinavian species of *Sarcoptes* is responsible for Norwegian scabies

See page 204 for answers

10. **Which of the following are signs of venous hypertension?**
    A Ulceration between the toes
    B Atrophie blanche
    C Cold feet
    D Lipodermatosclerosis
    E Pigmentation of the lower leg

11. **Which of the following are recognised causes of erythema nodosum?**
    A Streptococcal infection
    B Sarcoidosis
    C Systemic lupus erythematosus
    D Intravenous drug abuse
    E Inflammatory bowel disease

12. **Subepidermal blisters are seen in which of the following?**
    A Chicken pox
    B Pemphigus vulgaris
    C Epidermolysis bullosa simplex
    D Bullous pemphigoid
    E Dermatitis herpetiformis

13. **Which of the following are features of alopecia areata?**
    A A strong association with rheumatoid arthritis
    B Exclamation mark hairs
    C Increased incidence of organ-specific autoantibodies
    D A family history of alopecia areata
    E Eventual regrowth in all patients

14. **Which of the following may trigger urticaria?**
    A Heat
    B Cold
    C Aspirin
    D All of the above
    E None of the above

15. **Which of the following are recognized treatments for psoriasis?**
    A Dithranol
    B Vitamin D analogues
    C Streptokinase
    D Terbinafine
    E Infra-red radiation

16. **Which of the following are recognized treatments for acne in men?**
    A Oestrogens
    B Topical steroids
    C Topical erythromycin
    D Oral erythromycin
    E Oral isotretinoin

17. **Which of the following lesions have malignant potential?**
    A Mongolian blue spot
    B Seborrhoeic keratosis
    C Dermatofibroma
    D Solar (actinic) keratosis
    E Erythroplasia of Queyrat

18. **Which of the following are cutaneous features of systemic sclerosis?**
    A Calcinosis
    B Raynaud's phenomenon
    C Ecchymoses
    D Gottron's papules
    E Photosensitivity

19. **Onycholysis may be a sign of which of the following?**
    A Thyrotoxicosis
    B Myxoedema
    C Calcium deficiency
    D Lichen planus
    E Psoriasis

20. **Which of the following may lead to exfoliative dermatitis (erythroderma)?**
    A Lead poisoning
    B Cutaneous T-cell lymphoma
    C Psoriasis
    D Scurvy
    E Drug allergy

See page 204 for answers

abscess A localized collection of pus in a cavity formed by disintegration or necrosis of tissues, and usually caused by a microorganism.

acantholysis (Gk *akantha*—thorn and *lyein*—to loosen, free) Separation of epidermal keratinocytes resulting from loss of intercellular connections (desmosomes), causing the cells to become rounded and resulting in clefts. As occurs in *pemphigus* and *Darier's disease*.

acanthosis (Gk *akantha*—thorn, prickle) Increased thickness of the prickle-cell layer of the epidermis. As occurs in *psoriasis* and *lichenified eczema*.

acro- (Gk *akros*—outermost, extreme) Tip, extremity or top. As in *thyrotoxic acropachy*.

acrochordon Skin tag.

actinic (Gk *aktis, aktinos*—ray) Pertaining to rays or beams of light. As in *actinic keratosis*.

acuminate (L *acuminatus*—pointed, sharpened) Tapering or sharply pointed. As in *acuminate warts*.

agminate (L *agmen, agminis*—group) Grouped (of lesions).

alopecia (Gk *alōpekia*—a disease like the mange of foxes) Loss of hair.

angiokeratoma A vascular lesion in which dilatation of blood vessels is combined with hyperkeratosis.

anhidrosis Lack of sweating.

aphthae Painful ulcers of mucosae.

apocrine Relating to a gland which produces a secretion containing not only fluid but also cellular granules.

aquagenic Caused by contact with water. As in *aquagenic pruritus*.

arborizing (L *arbor*—tree) Branching, as of a tree. For example, *arborizing telangiectasia*.

atopy (atopic) Predisposing to the development of diseases associated with excessive IgE antibody formation.

atrophy A wasting or shrinking of a cell, tissue or organ.

Auspitz sign A sign described by an Austrian dermatologist that features punctate haemorrhage from superficial dermal capillaries upon removal of scale in psoriasis.

balanitis Inflammation of the glans penis.

balanoposthitis Inflammation of the glans penis and prepuce.

balsam of Peru Mixture of oil and resin obtained from the tree *Myroxolon pereirae*. Used as an antiseptic.

Beau's lines Transverse depressions on the nail plates associated with growth arrest during serious illness.

Becker's naevus Hairy, pigmented epidermal naevus occurring on the shoulder area.

Behçet's syndrome Named after a Turkish dermatologist. The main features of this syndrome are orogenital ulceration and iritis.

berloque dermatitis (Fr *berloque*—a pendant) A streaky form of pigmented photodermatitis occurring on the neck and caused by psoralens, usually bergamot oil, in perfumes.

Besnier's prurigo An alternative name for atopic dermatitis.

Blaschko's lines A system of lines whose pattern is followed by many naevoid skin conditions.

blepharitis Inflammation of the eyelid.

boil Colloquial term for a furuncle.

Bowen's disease Epidermal squamous cell carcinoma *in situ*.

bromhidrosis (Gk *bromos*—stench and *hidrōs*—sweat) Foul-smelling sweat, usually resulting from bacterial action on axillary apocrine secretions.

bulla (pl. bullae) (L *bulla*—a bubble) A blister. A fluid-filled bleb.

burrow A tunnel in the epidermis occupied by the scabies mite.

callus (callosity) Localized thickening of the skin, particularly the horny layer, in response to repeated pressure or friction.

Campbell de Morgan spots Cherry angiomata. Small, age-related vascular lesions. Campbell de Morgan was a British physician.

canities (L *canities*—grey hair) Greying or whitening of hair.

carbuncle A deep infection of a group of contiguous hair follicles with *Staphylococcus aureus*, resulting in the formation of a multiloculated abscess.

Casal's necklace An area of erythema and pigmentation around the neck, occurring in pellagra.

cheilitis (Gk *cheilos*—lip) Inflammation of the lips.

cheiro- (Gk *cheiros*—hand) Meaning hand.

cheiropompholyx A blistering eruption of the hands.

cheloid Alternative spelling of keloid.

chilblain A lesion resulting from a vascular response to cold. Also called *pernio, perniosis*.

chloasma Patchy pigmentation of the face. Also known as *melasma*.

chrysiasis Deposition of gold in the tissues.

clavus A corn.

colophony Rosin obtained from pine trees. Many uses, but perhaps best known as a component of adhesive plasters.

comedo A plug in a pilosebaceous follicle.

condyloma (pl. condylomata) A wart-like tumour or growth. Usually applied to genital warts (*condylomata acuminata*) and secondary syphilitic lesions in the anogenital region (*condylomata lata*).

conglobata (L *conglobare*—to gather into a rounded form) Clumped or clustered. As used in a severe type of acne (*acne conglobata*).

craquelé Cracked. Resembling crazy paving. As in *eczema craquelé*.

Crowe's sign Axillary freckling in neurofibromatosis.

CRST (CREST) syndrome Most common form of systemic sclerosis. Calcinosis, *R*aynaud's phe-

nomenon, *E*sophageal involvement (American spelling), *S*clerodactyly, *T*elangiectasia.

cyst Any closed cavity or sac with a lining and containing fluid or other material.

dandruff A popular term for *pityriasis capitis*.

Darier's sign Named after a famous French dermatologist, this is the occurrence of wealing on rubbing lesions of urticaria pigmentosa.

Dennie–Morgan folds Prominent folds in lower eyelid skin seen in atopic individuals.

depilation (epilation) Removal of hair.

depilatory Any agent used to remove or destroy hair.

dermabrasion Removal of skin lesions by a variety of abrading devices such as a rapidly turning wire brush.

dermatoglyphics Epidermal ridge patterns on hands and feet.

dhobi itch Colloquial term used for any itchy condition affecting the groins/pubic region, particularly ringworm. A dhobi is an Indian washerman.

diascopy Examination of a skin lesion by applying firm pressure over it with a glass slide. Used particularly to demonstrate 'apple-jelly' nodules in lupus vulgaris.

dyschromatosis Abnormal pigmentation

dyskeratosis Abnormal keratinization.

dysmorphophobia A disturbance in perception of body image.

ecchymosis A bruise

ectasia Dilatation of a duct or vessel. As in *lymphangiectasia*.

ecthyma A heavily crusted, deep-seated pyogenic infection.

eczema An inflammatory skin reaction characterized by itching, redness, vesiculation, exudation and crusting.

ephelis A freckle.

epidermotropism Movement towards the epidermis.

epiloia Derived from **epi**lepsy, **lo**w intelligence and adenoma sebaceum. An alternative name for tuberous sclerosis complex.

erysipelas A superficial form of cellulitis caused by haemolytic streptococci.

erythema (Gk *erythēma*—redness)   Redness of the skin.

furuncle   Localized pyogenic inflammation in a hair follicle. Also known as a *boil*.

glabrous   Smooth, hairless.

Gottron's papules   Erythematous papules overlying finger joints in dermatomyositis.

Hansen's disease   Leprosy. Hansen was a Norwegian bacteriologist who first demonstrated *Mycobacterium leprae*.

herpetiform   Grouped vesicles resembling herpes.

hirsutism (L *hirsutus*—shaggy)   The growth of hair in women in the male sexual pattern.

hives   Popular US term for urticaria.

ichthyosis (Gk *ichthys*—fish)   A group of disorders of keratinization characterized by scaling likened to fish skin.

intertrigo   Inflammation of apposed skin surfaces such as groins, axillae and inframammary regions.

Kaposi's varicelliform eruption   Named after a famous Hungarian-born dermatologist, this is disseminated infection with herpes simplex or vaccinia virus in atopic individuals.

keloid (cheloid)   Excessive scar tissue formation extending beyond the original area of injury.

kerion (GK *kērion*—honeycomb)   A severe inflammatory response to the presence of fungal infection, usually of animal origin, on hair-bearing areas.

Koebner (Köbner) phenomenon   The provocation of skin lesions by trauma, seen in *psoriasis*, *lichen planus* and *vitiligo*. Köbner was a German dermatologist.

Koenen's tumours   Periungual fibromata in tuberous sclerosis complex.

koilonychia (Gk *koilos*—hollow and *onychos*—nail)   Spoon-shaped nails, typically a feature of severe iron deficiency.

Langerhans cells   Epidermal dendritic cells, characterized by the presence of racquet-shaped 'Birbeck' granules, acting as specialized antigen-presenting cells.

Lassar's paste   Zinc oxide paste with salicylic acid.

lentigo   A pigmented macule with an increased number of melanocytes at the dermo-epidermal junction.

leukoderma (leukoderma) (Gk *leukos*—white and *derma*—skin)   Lack of normal pigmentation of the skin. Non-specific term which in lay usage is often applied to vitiligo.

leukoplakia   Persistent white patches on mucous membranes.

lichen (Gk *leichēn*—a tree moss)   Resembling a tree moss/lichen. As in *lichen planus*.

licheniform   Resembling lichen planus.

livedo (L *livere*—to be blue or bluish)   A cyanotic discoloration of the skin that follows the cutaneous vascular network.

lupus (L *lupus*—wolf)   Applied to lesions that involve tissue damage likened to the gnawing of a wolf. For example, *lupus vulgaris* and *lupus erythematosus*.

Lyell's syndrome   Toxic epidermal necrolysis.

Lyme disease   Lyme is a town in Connecticut where the association between ticks, a spirochaete (*Borrelia burgdorferi*), and an arthropathy was first established.

madarosis   Loss of eyelashes.

Madura foot   Named after a town in southern India, it is another name for a mycetoma.

Mees' lines   Transverse white bands on the nails in arsenic and thallium poisoning.

melasma   Patchy hyperpigmentation of the face. Also known as *chloasma*.

milium (pl. milia) (L *milium*—millet seed)   Tiny white keratin cyst.

Mohs' micrographic surgery   Named after the US surgeon who developed the technique, this is a method of layer by layer excision of tumours with histological assessment of excision margins.

morbilliform   Measles-like.

Muehrke's striae   White bands on the nail occurring in severe hypoalbuminaemia.

myiasis (Gk *myia*—a fly)   Invasion of tissues by fly larvae.

naevus   A localized cutaneous malformation involving either an excess or relative deficiency of any of the normal cutaneous structures. A cutaneous hamartoma.

necrobiosis Physiological or normal cell death in the midst of living tissue. As in *necrobiosis lipoidica*.

necrolysis (Gk *nekros*—dead and *lyein*—to loosen, free) Separation of dead tissue. As in the epidermis in toxic epidermal necrolysis.

Nikolsky's sign Separation of the epidermis produced by firm sliding pressure of the finger. Occurs in *pemphigus* and *toxic epidermal necrolysis*. Nikolsky was a Russian dermatologist.

nitidus Glistening, shiny. As in *lichen nitidus*.

nummular (L *nummulus* dim. of *nummus*—coin) In the shape of a coin. Discoid.

onychogryphosis (Gk *onychos*—nail and *grypos*—curved, hooked) Thickening and overcurvature of the nail resembling a ram's horn.

onychoschizia (Gk *onychos*—nail and *schizein*—to cleave or split) Splitting of the nail plate into layers.

ophiasis (Gk *ophis*—snake) Snake-like. A pattern of alopecia areata affecting the scalp margin.

pachyonychia (Gk *pachys*—thick and *onychos*—nail) Abnormally thick nails.

papilloma A nipple-like projection from the skin.

Pautrier's abscess Focal collection of lymphocytes in the epidermis in mycosis fungoides.

peau d'orange A dimpling appearance of the skin simulating orange peel. Seen in carcinoma of the breast.

pellagra A disorder caused by dietary deficiency of niacin (nicotinic acid).

perlèche (Fr *pourlécher*—to lick one's lips) Angular cheilitis.

pernio (perniosis) (L *pernio*—chilblain) Chilblain.

petechia (pl. petechiae) A punctate haemorrhagic spot.

photo- (Gk *phōtos*—light) Pertaining to light.

phyto- (Gk *phyton*—plant, tree) Pertaining to plants.

pityriasis (L *pityriasi*—scurf, from Gk *pityron*—bran) A branny scaling of the skin. As in *pityriasis versicolor*.

poikiloderma (Gk *poikilos*—mottled, dappled and *derma*—skin) Dappled pigmentation, usually associated with telangiectasia and atrophy.

poliosis (Gk *poliosis*—becoming grey) Localized patches of white hair. As in *piebaldism*.

pompholyx (Gk *pompholyx*—a bubble) Acute vesiculobullous eruption on hands (cheiro-) and feet (podo-).

Prurigo (L *prurigo*—itching) Term used in some conditions associated with itching, including *nodular prurigo* and *Besnier's prurigo* (atopic dermatitis).

psoriasiform Resembling psoriasis.

psoriasis (Gk *psōriasis*, from *psōra*—itch, mange, scab) A chronic skin disease typically manifesting scaly plaques.

pterygium (Gk *pterygion*—a little wing) Used to denote a web or fold of skin, for example *pterygium colli* (webbed neck in Turner's syndrome) and the tissue encroaching on the nail apparatus in lichen planus of the nails.

pyoderma Generic name for any purulent skin condition.

reticulate (L *reticulatus*—net-shaped) In a net-like pattern.

rhinophyma (Gk *rhis, rhinos*—nose and *phyma*—inflamed swelling) Connective tissue and sebaceous gland hypertrophy of the nose as a feature of rosacea in men.

sclerosis (Gk *sklēros*—hard) Thickening, induration.

shagreen (Fr *peau de chagrin*) Resembling shark skin or untanned leather with a rough surface. As in *shagreen patches*—connective tissue naevi on the back in tuberous sclerosis complex.

shingles (L *cingulum*—girdle, belt) Colloquial term for herpes zoster.

Sister Joseph's nodule Umbilical metastasis from intra-abdominal neoplasm. Named after Sister Mary Joseph who worked with Dr William James Mayo and is said to have pointed out its significance to him.

squame (L *squama*—a scale of a fish or serpent) A scale.

sycosis (Gk *sykon*—a fig) Deep inflammation of hair follicles. As in *sycosis barbae*—inflammation of the beard area.

telangiectasia (telangiectasis) (Gk *telos*—end, *angeion*—vessel and *ektasis*—dilatation) Dilatation of small blood vessels.

tinea (L *tinea*—a gnawing worm) A dermatophyte fungal infection.

trich-, tricho- (Gk *trichos*—hair) Relating to hair. As in *trichology*.

trichotillomania Compulsive hair pulling.

trichophytide A rash provoked by an immunological response to a fungal infection. For example, pompholyx on the hands provoked by a severe inflammatory fungal infection on the foot.

verruca In common use referring to a plantar wart, but in fact a term applicable to a wart at any site.

weal This is the correct spelling. A transient, raised, itchy lesion occurring in urticaria and dermographism.

whitlow Infection of finger pulp. As in *herpetic whitlow*.

Wickham's striae Pattern of lace-like greyish-white lines on the surface of lesions of lichen planus. Louis Wickham was a French dermatologist.

Wood's light A source of filtered ultraviolet light that is used to demonstrate fluorescence caused by certain organisms. For example, *Microsporum canis* [tinea capitis] (yellow-green) and *Corynebacterium minutissimum* [erythrasma] (coral pink).

xerosis (Gk *xeros*—dry) Dryness.

Answers to multiple choice questions

1. A, C, D, E
2. A
3. B, C, E
4. A, B, C, E
5. B, C, E
6. A, B, E
7. A
8. B, C
9. A, D
10. B, D, E

11. A, B, E
12. D, E
13. B, C, D
14. D
15. A, B
16. C, D, E
17. D, E
18. A, B
19. A, E
20. B, C, E

Index

Page numbers in *italics* indicate illustrations that are not on the same page as the relevant text.

Chemical synthesis of advanced ceramic materials

David Segal

Materials Chemistry Department, Harwell Laboratory, Oxfordshire

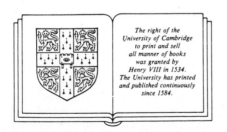

The right of the
University of Cambridge
to print and sell
all manner of books
was granted by
Henry VIII in 1534.
The University has printed
and published continuously
since 1584.

Cambridge University Press

Cambridge

New York   Port Chester   Melbourne   Sydney

Published by the Press Syndicate of the University of Cambridge
The Pitt Building, Trumpington Street, Cambridge CB2 1RP
40 West 20th Street, New York, NY 10011–4211, USA
10 Stamford Road, Oakleigh, Melbourne 3166, Australia

First published 1989
First paperback edition 1991

Printed in Great Britain at the University Press, Cambridge

British Library cataloguing in publication data

Segal, David
Chemical synthesis of advanced ceramic
materials
1. Materials.   Ceramics.   Synthesis
I. Title   II. Series
620.1′4

Library of Congress cataloguing in publication data

Segal, David, 1950–
Chemical synthesis of advanced ceramic material / David Segal.
    p.   cm.
Bibliography: p.
Includes index.
ISBN 0 521 35436 6
1. Ceramics.   I. Title.
TP815.S465 1989
666—dc 19   88-27537 CIP

ISBN 0 521 35436 6 hardback
ISBN 0 521 42418 6 paperback

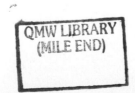

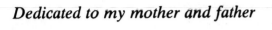

Dedicated to my mother and father

Contents

Contents

Contents

Preface

Advanced ceramic materials have attracted increasing attention throughout the 1980s from many disciplines including chemistry, physics,
metallurgy and materials science and this multidisciplinary approach
is illustrated by the diverse range of journals and conferences where information is disseminated. In addition the discovery of high-temperature
ceramic superconductors in 1986 has raised the profile of advanced
ceramics activities not only within the scientific community but also
among the general public. Attendance at conferences and surveys of
scientific literature show that chemical synthetic methods have played an
increasing role, over the past fifteen years, in improving the properties of
ceramic materials. Books concerned with fabrication and physical
properties of ceramics do not, in my opinion, highlight chemical aspects
of ceramic preparations which are not the principal interest of physical,
organic and inorganic chemistry textbooks.

My discussions with undergraduate and postgraduate students in
chemistry and materials science as well as university lecturers and those
in industry concerned with research into and manufacture of advanced
ceramics produced two conclusions. Firstly, there did not seem to be a
short volume available which acted as a bridge between pure chemistry
and conventional ceramic studies such as fabrication. Also, although
scientific publications and conference proceedings proliferate it was not
obvious how a comprehensive view of the rapid inroads chemistry is
making into ceramic synthesis could be obtained. I see this book as that
bridge between pure chemical and conventional ceramic studies. I have
included a chapter on fabrication for continuity but this is not the main
theme. I have not discussed the mechanisms and structures of all
reactions and materials described here, or listed 'recipes' for ceramic

synthesis. What I have attempted to show is the role chemistry has in the synthesis of advanced ceramic materials but, at all times, synthetic routes are related to the desired ceramic properties for materials in the form of powders, fibre, coatings or monoliths made on the laboratory and industrial scale. All branches of chemistry contribute to advanced ceramic development but three areas occur repeatedly throughout this book, namely colloid chemistry, homogeneous nucleation processes and chemistry at the organic–inorganic interface.

Finally, a paragraph on acknowledgements. I thank authors and copyright owners in Europe, Japan, Australia and The United States of America for giving permission to reproduce their photographs in this book. I am indebted to staff of the Harwell Library who obtained numerous scientific publications for me while line diagrams were drawn in the Tracing Office at Harwell. Anita Harvey typed the manuscript; and lastly an acknowledgement to my employer, The United Kingdom Atomic Energy Authority for permission to publish this book.

Harwell Laboratory   David Segal

Symbols

N	Avogadro number
h	Planck's constant
k	Boltzmann constant
e	Electronic charge
c	Ionic strength
z	Ion valency
$\%$	Percentage
T	Absolute temperature
T_c	Superconducting transition or critical temperature
E	Young's modulus
S	Tensile fracture strength
$2C$	Crack length
C_1	BET constant
S_A	Surface area
D	Diffusion coefficient
D_c	Crystallite dimension
K	Equilibrium constant
K_{IC}	Fracture toughness
K^*	Constant in Scherrer equation (A.3)
G	Gravitational constant
η	Liquid viscosity
κ	Reciprocal double layer thickness
Q	Scattering vector
Ω	Angular rotational velocity
R, R'	Alkyl chain
R^*	Reflectivity at near normal incidence
R_G	Gas constant
λ	Wavelength
L	Nucleation rate per unit volume
I, I_0	Scattered intensity
$P(\phi)$	Shape factor
ϕ	Angle between incident and scattered radiation
V_L	London energy between two atoms
V_A	van der Waals – London energy for macroscopic bodies
V_R	Electrostatic energy of repulsion
V_S	Free energy due to adsorbed layer overlap
V_T	Total potential energy between particles
θ_B	Bragg angle

Symbols

$\theta_{1/2}$	Pure diffraction broadening at half-peak height
θ	Contact angle at solid-air-liquid interface
I_R	Rayleigh scattered intensity
I_{RG}	Rayleigh–Gans scattered intensity
ψ_0	Surface charge
ν_0	Ground-state electron vibrational frequency
α	Static atomic polarizability
λ^*	$= 3h\nu_0\alpha^2/4$

$A, A_1,$ A_2, A_{12}	Hamaker constant
a	Sphere radius
H_0	Separation of spheres or flat plates at closest approach
x	$= H_0/2a$
q	Number of molecules per unit volume of material
ε_0	Permittivity of vacuum
ε	Relative permittivity of medium
l	Side length of a cube
l_0	Sample to detector distance
l_1	Sedimentation distance
l_2	Distance between particle and axis of rotation
l_3	Radius of rotation for particles
$n_0, n_1, n_2,$ n_p, n_m	Refractive index
n	Number of molecules in critical cluster
$\Delta G'_n$	Free energy of formation for critical cluster
r	Distance between atoms
r_p	Pore radius
r_d	Radius of liquid droplet
r_g	Radius of gyration
r_n	Critical radius of cluster
b, f, g, j, δ	Number of moles
$t_{1/2}$	Half-life

$t, t_1, t_2,$ t_3, t_c, τ	Time
ρ, ρ_p, ρ_1	Density
γ	Surface tension of liquid
γ'	Surface energy
Δ_p	Capillary pressure
$p_F, p_G,$ p_J	Partial gas pressures
p^0	Saturation vapour pressure
p'	Vapour pressure
p	Gas pressure
M_w	Molecular weight
$\bar{M}_w$	Weight average molecular weight
$\bar{M}_n$	Number average molecular weight
h_c	Coating thickness
C_x, C_0	Concentration of solute or reactant
C_s	Saturated solute concentration

Symbols

C_{SS}	Supersaturated solute concentration
N_p	Number of particles
β	Overall growth coefficient for droplets
v	Molar volume of liquid phase
v_l	Volume of molecule in liquid phase
v_a	Adsorbate volume at a specified relative pressure
v_m	Adsorbate volume for monolayer coverage per unit mass of solid
m	Mass of a molecule
m_d	Volume of a diffusing vacancy
M	Metal

1 Introduction: the variety of ceramic systems

1.1 Introduction

The international advanced ceramics industry is concerned with basic research and ceramic fabrication as well as manufacture of powders and fibres while the success of research can be measured by its application to large-scale economic production of ceramics which function in particular working environments. Advanced ceramic materials are defined in this introductory chapter and their variety and uses are explained. The ceramics industry is large and an indication of its volume production and monetary value is also given here. Finally, the recent discovery of high-temperature oxide superconductors has had a tremendous impact on worldwide ceramic activities and a section is included on the properties and potential applications of these advanced ceramic materials.

1.2 From traditional to advanced ceramics

Ceramics are the group of non-metallic inorganic solids and their use by man dates from the time of ancient civilisations. In fact, the word ceramic is of Greek origin and its translation (keramos) means potter's earth. Traditional ceramics are those derived from naturally occurring raw materials and include clay-based products such as tableware and sanitaryware as well as structural claywares like bricks and pipes. Also in this category are cements, glasses and refractories. Examples of the latter are chrome–magnesite refractories used in the steel-making industry and derived from magnesite ($MgCO_3$) and chrome ore. Advanced ceramics are developed from chemical synthetic routes or from naturally occurring materials that have been highly refined. A variety of names has been used to describe ceramic systems. Hence, advanced ceramics are also called engineering ceramics whereas the phrases 'special', 'fine' and 'technical' have all been used in connection with these materials. When their use depends on mechanical behaviour, advanced ceramics are sometimes referred to as structural components whereas electroceramics are a class of advanced ceramic whose application relies on electrical and magnetic properties. Books by Norton (1968) and Shaw (1972) contain further details on traditional ceramics whereas Morrell (1985) has described the classification of ceramic systems.

1.3   Structural and refractory applications of engineering ceramics

Structural components derived from engineering ceramics are used as monoliths, coatings and composites in conjunction with or as replacements for metals when applications rely on mechanical behaviour of the ceramics and their refractory properties, that is chemical resistance to the working environment. Physical properties of ceramics and metals are compared in table 1.1 some of their magnitudes are shown in tables 1.2 and 1.3. Nickel superalloys are currently the main high-temperature materials for components such as combustors in gas turbine engines (Meetham, 1986). They have melting points around 1573 K and a maximum working temperature near 1300 K. Cast iron parts in reciprocating (i.e. petrol and diesel) engines have properties shown in table 1.3. Compared with metals, ceramics are generally more resistant to oxidation, corrosion, creep and wear in addition to being better thermal insulators. They have higher melting points (table 1.4) and greater strength than superalloys at elevated temperature so that a major potential application, particularly for silicon nitride, is in gas turbine and reciprocating engines where operating temperatures higher than attainable with metals can result in greater efficiencies. This enhanced strength is shown in figure 1.1 for hot-pressed silicon nitride (HPSN), hot-pressed silicon carbide (HPSC), hot isostatically pressed silicon nitride (HIPSN), sintered silicon nitride (SSN), sintered silicon carbide (SSC), reaction-bonded silicon nitride (RBSN) and reaction-bonded silicon carbide (RBSC). Although ceramics offer improvements in engine efficiency, incorporation of silicon nitride over the past three decades has been slow, mainly because of the difficulty in reproducible fabrication of dense components to close dimensional tolerances.

Silicon nitride occurs in two phases, the α and the β forms. The β form, whose structure is shown in figure 1.2, consists of SiN_4 tetrahedra joined together by sharing corners in a three-dimensional network. It is

Structural and refractory applications

Table 1.1. *Relative properties of ceramics and metals (AE Development, 1985)*

Property	Ceramics	Metals	Ratio, property of ceramics: property of metal
Ductility	Very low	High	$(0.001–0.01):1$
Density	Low	High	$0.5:1$
Fracture toughness	Low	High	$(0.01–0.1):1$
Young's modulus	High	Low	$(1–3):1$
Hardness	High	Low	$(3–10):1$
Thermal expansion	Low	High	$(0.1–0.3):1$
Thermal conductivity	Low	High	$(0.05–0.2):1$
Electrical resistance	High	Low	$(10^6–10^{10}):1$

Table 1.2. *Physical properties for alloys, oxide and non-oxide ceramics (Briscoe, 1986)*

Material	Specific gravity $(kg\,m^{-3})$	Thermal expansion coefficient $(10^{-6}\,K^{-1})$	Thermal conductivity $(W\,m^{-1}\,K^{-1})$
Alumina	4000	9	20
Toughened zirconia polycrystals	5800	10	2
Sintered silicon carbide	3100	4.5	40
Sintered silicon nitride	3100	3.2	12
Hot-pressed silicon nitride	3100	3.1	30
Window glass	2200	9	1
Aluminium alloys	2800	22	146
Nimonic superalloys	8500	15	16

possible to replace silicon by aluminium and maintain charge neutrality in the crystal lattice by substitution of nitrogen with oxygen. The resulting solid solutions in the Si–Al–O–N system are known as β'-sialons (K. H. Jack, 1986) whose structures are identical with β-Si$_3$N$_4$ over the composition range $Si_{6-b}Al_bO_bN_{8-b}$ $(0<b<4)$. They exhibit mechanical behaviour similar to β-Si$_3$N$_4$ and have some features of aluminium oxide. However, in contrast with Al$_2$O$_3$, which consists of six-coordinated Al,

Introduction: the variety of ceramic systems

Table 1.3. *Mechanical properties of cast irons, oxide and non-oxide ceramics (Lackey et al., 1987)*

Material	Young's modulus GPa	Fracture toughness (MPa m$^{1/2}$)	Fracture strength at room temperature MPa
Alumina	380	2.7–4.2	276–1034
Partially stabilised zirconia	205	8–9 at 293 K	
		6–6.5 at 723 K	600–700
		5 at 1073 K	
Sintered silicon carbide	207–483	4.8 at 300 K	96–520
		2.6–5.0 at 1273 K	
Sintered silicon nitride	304	5.3	414–650
Hot-pressed silicon nitride	304	4.1–6.0	700–1000
Glass ceramics	83–138	2.4	70–350
Pyrex glass	70	0.75	69
Cast irons	83–211	37–45	90–1186

Table 1.4. *Melting point and maximum working temperatures of ceramics (Lay, 1983)*

Material	Melting point or decomposition temperature/K	Maximum working temperature/K	
		In oxidising atmosphere	In reducing atmosphere
Alumina	2323	2173	2173
Stabilised zirconia	2823	2473	
Silicon carbide	2873	1923	2593
Boron carbide	2723	873	2273
Tungsten carbide	3023	823	2273
Reaction-bonded silicon nitride	2173	1473	2143
Boron nitride	2573	1473	2473
Titanium diboride	3253	1073	>2273

β'-sialon contains Al that is four-coordinated by oxygen and this results in an enhanced Al–O bond strength compared with the oxide. Unlike Si_3N_4, β'-sialons can be densified readily by pressureless sintering and they have been put into commercial production by Lucas Cookson

Syalon Limited. Syalon components shown in figure 1.3 include auto-
motive parts such as valves, valve guides and seats, tappets, rocker
inserts and precombustion chambers in addition to weld shrouds,
location pins, extrusion dies, tube drawing dies and plugs.

Aluminium titanate is used as port liners in some automobile engines
because its low thermal conductivity (2 W m^{-1} K^{-1}) reduces heat flow to
the cylinder block and hence the amount of cooling required. Glass
ceramics have applications (table 2.1) in cooking utensils, tableware,
heat exchangers, vacuum tube components and missile radomes.
Partially stabilised zirconia was developed in 1975 at the Australian
Commonwealth Scientific & Industrial Research Organisation (CSIRO)
and is nowadays manufactured by Nilcra-PSZ Limited. This material is
particularly suited for withstanding mechanical and thermal shock
because of its high fracture toughness (table 1.3). Examples are dies for

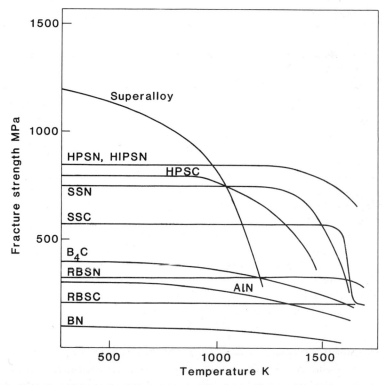

Figure 1.1. Variation of strength with temperature for non-oxide ceramics
(Heinrich, 1985).

extrusion of copper and aluminium tubes, diesel engine cam follower faces, valve guides, cylinder liners and piston caps, wear and corrosion-resistant nozzles in papermaking equipment, wear resistant inserts such as tabletting dies as well as scissors and knives.

Not all ceramic components require high-temperature strength. The high Young's modulus (550 GPa) of titanium diboride, TiB_2, makes it useful for armour plating (Knoch, 1987) whereas ceramics are suitable materials in seals because of their chemical resistance (table 1.5). Hence sintered silicon carbide is used for mechanical seals and sliding bearings whereas boron nitride, which is not wetted by glass and liquid metals, constitutes break rings in the horizontal continuous casting process for steels. Boron carbide, a harder ceramic than SiC, is suited to wear-resistant applications such as grit blasting nozzles whereas Si_3N_4 is also

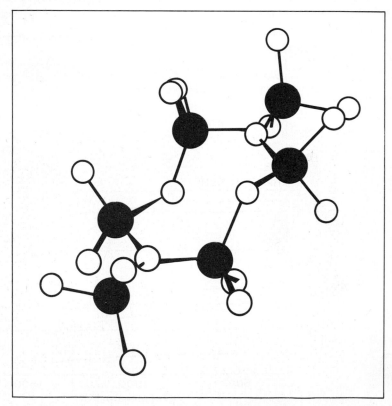

Figure 1.2. Crystal structure of β-Si_3N_4 and β'-$(Si,Al)_3(O,N)_4$. ●, metal atom, ○, non-metal atom (K. H. Jack, 1986).